VEGAN RECIPES IN 30 MINUTES

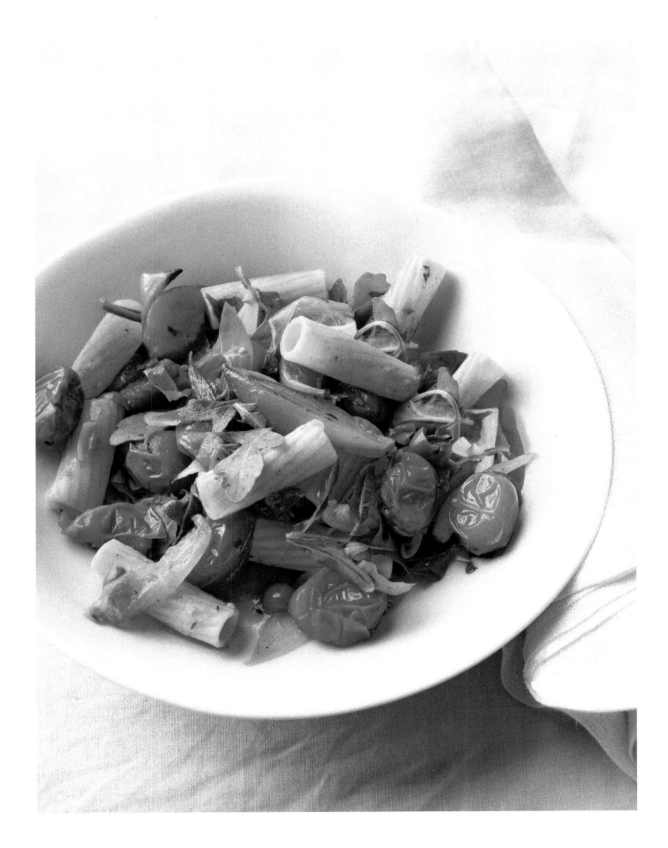

VEGAN
RECIPES IN
30 MINUTES

A Vegan Cookbook with
106 Quick & Easy Recipes

SHASTA
PRESS

CONTENTS

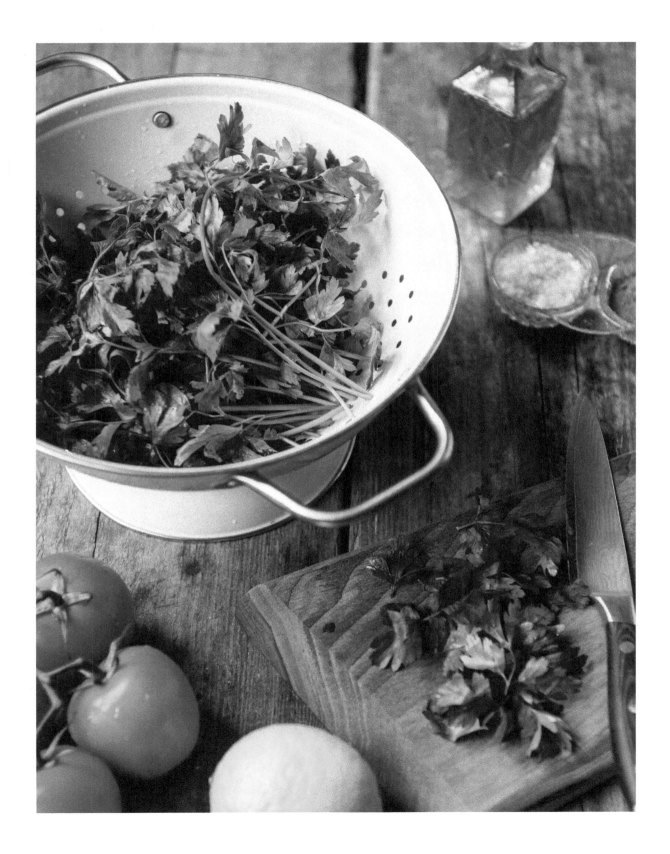

INTRODUCTION

Welcome to *Vegan Recipes in 30 Minutes*. If you lead a busy life and have minimal time to prepare meals, then this book is for you. *Vegan Recipes in 30 Minutes* provides busy vegan home cooks with recipes that:

- Taste great.
- Are budget-friendly.
- Use ten ingredients or fewer (not counting salt, pepper, or optional ingredients).
- Require fewer than 15 minutes of prep time.
- Can be on your table in fewer than 30 minutes.
- Use healthy ingredients you can find at your local grocery store or farm stand.
- Minimize the use of processed ingredients.
- Are easy to prepare.
- Rely on simple cooking techniques.
- Don't require special equipment.

Quick and Easy

In today's busy world, home cooks need recipes for budget-friendly, healthy, and delicious meals they can prepare quickly. At the beginning of each recipe, you will find both preparation time and cooking time as an indication of approximately how long the recipe will take.

Fresh, Natural Ingredients

Many people, fearing the amount of time it takes to prepare homemade vegan dishes, turn to processed foods. These foods, while technically vegan, aren't always the healthiest choices. The convenience of such foods comes at a cost, both nutritionally and financially. Processed foods often contain additives, preservatives, and chemicals that don't support vibrant good health.

The recipes in this book rely on affordable, fresh, natural ingredients you can find at your local grocery store or farm stand, such as fruits, vegetables, whole grains, legumes, nuts, seeds, herbs, and spices. These ingredients are real, whole foods that nourish your body naturally.

In many of the recipes, you can substitute seasonal local produce to save money. You can replace fresh ingredients with affordable frozen and canned foods in many cases. Possible substitutions for ingredients are noted in parentheses on ingredient lists for each recipe.

Vegan Cooking on a Budget

The recipes in this book also keep your budget in mind. Along with discovering recipes that use inexpensive and easy-to-source ingredients, you'll also find tips to help you save both time and money, such as a list of affordable pantry staples; methods for storing foods and ingredients so they last longer; and healthy, time-saving prepared foods you can substitute for fresh.

Simple Instructions

Good cooking doesn't require complicated techniques. In fact, the recipes in this book have been designed with simplicity in mind, using straightforward, easy cooking techniques you've most likely already mastered. The recipes also contain ten or fewer ingredients (excluding salt, pepper, and optional ingredients). They are designed for busy people who want to eat fresh, affordable, delicious, and healthy vegan foods.

Variety

These recipes are also designed to keep meal and snack time interesting, providing a variety of flavors and textures. Along with delicious main dishes, you'll also find international foods, easy-to-make sandwiches and soups, quick breakfasts, tasty sides, and mouthwatering desserts.

Get Cooking!

With these simple, quick, easy-to-follow recipes, you'll be inspired to step into the kitchen and feed your family delicious homemade vegan meals.

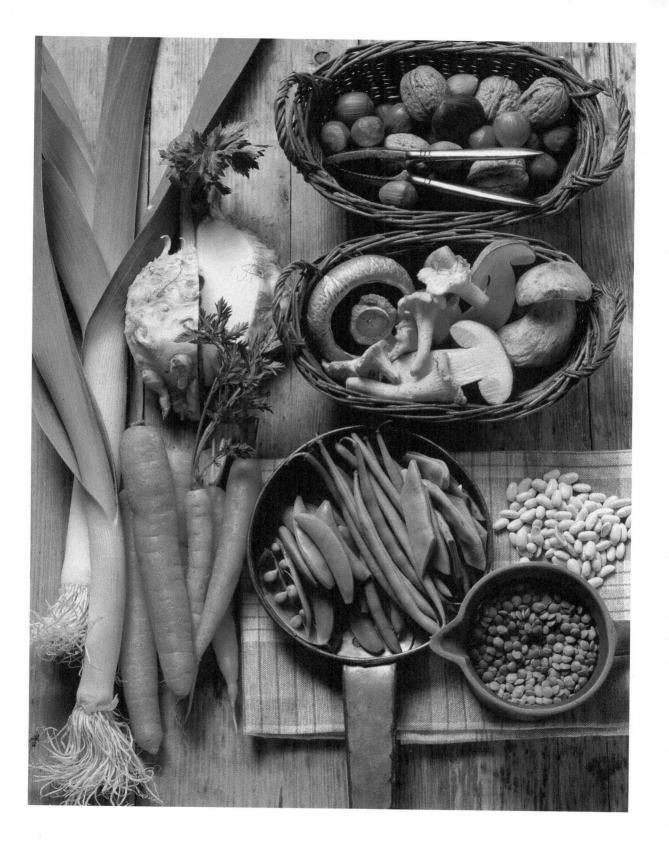

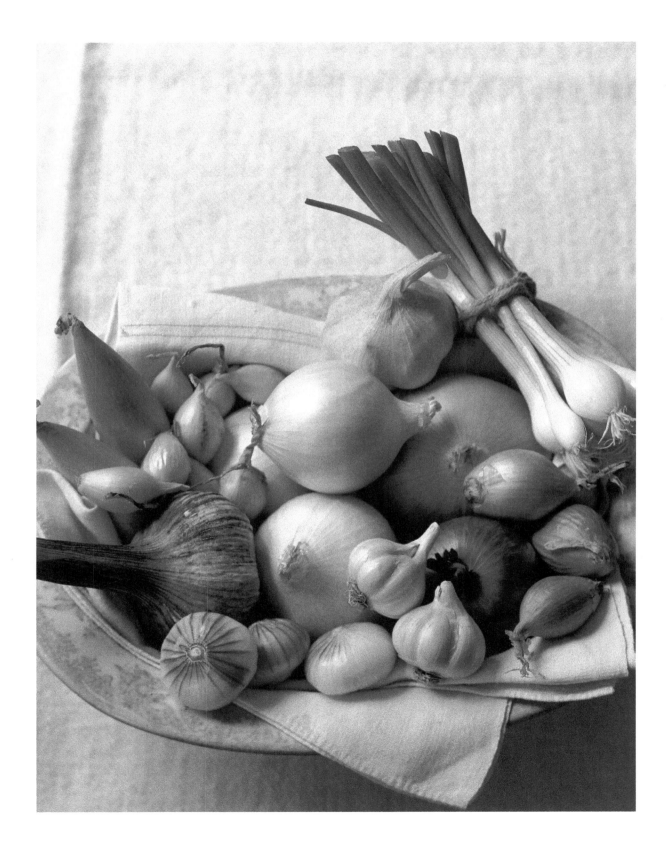

1

Veganism Explained

Veganism is not just another newfangled diet or passing fad. Plant-based and animal product–free diets have been around for centuries. Even the term "vegan" has been in circulation for decades. In the 1940s, several members of England's then nearly one-hundred-year-old Vegetarian Society split off to form their own organization that focused on a strictly plant-based diet that eschewed all animal-derived foods. These strict vegetarians chose the name "vegan" because, as one of the founding members of the first Vegan Society, Donald Watson, said, "veganism starts with vegetarianism and carries it through to its logical conclusion."

A vegan diet can be defined as a "total vegetarian" diet, meaning one that is entirely plant-based and omits all animal products, including meat, eggs, dairy, honey, gelatin, and other products that come from animals. Vegans eat a plant-based diet of vegetables, grains, legumes, fruits, nuts, and seeds.

Veganism, however, is much more than a diet. It is a way of life. Those who choose a vegan lifestyle not only eat plant-based foods but also choose not to purchase products made from leather, wool, silk, and down, including cosmetics and soaps that contain animal products or are tested on animals.

Why We Eat Vegan

While there are many reasons why people choose veganism—allergies, specific health concerns, and personal preference, among others—one of the main drives is a desire for a "cruelty-free" lifestyle that avoids exploiting animals and seeks to create a more humane society. Choosing to eat only plant-based foods is a decisive way to reduce animal suffering. And if your decision to become a vegan influences others to do the same, the effect is exponential.

Being vegan also helps the environment, since raising animals for food requires vital resources such as food and water, and in many cases, trees need to be razed to make room for ranches. Animal waste also contaminates the soil, air, and water. So great is the damage done to the environment by the meat industry that the Union of Concerned Scientists considers meat eating to be one of the biggest environmental hazards we face today, second only to our reliance on fossil-fueled vehicles.

Another popular reason for adopting a vegan diet is good health. A well-balanced vegan diet can be extremely healthy since it includes plenty of fruit, vegetables, whole grains, nuts, and seeds, making it rich in vitamins, antioxidants, and fiber.

Furthermore, by eating only plant-based foods, you automatically eliminate cholesterol and unhealthy saturated fats. Adhering to a well-balanced vegan diet can decrease the risk of developing many diseases, including diabetes, heart disease, stroke, and some types of cancer.

Vegans tend to be thinner and fitter than their meat- and/or dairy-eating counterparts, too. Just look at all the glamorous celebrities who have chosen this lifestyle: Ellen DeGeneres, Shania Twain, Casey Affleck, Tobey Maguire, Alicia Silverstone, Kristen Bell, Alyssa Milano, Joss Stone, Anne Hathaway, Michelle Pfeiffer, and Carrie Underwood, to name a few.

Finally, eating a plant-based diet is economical. The diet is centered on whole grains, legumes, fruits, vegetables, nuts, and seeds—all of which are generally much less expensive than meat or dairy products, especially when purchased in season.

Guidelines and Rules for Eating Vegan

A vegan diet can be a very healthy way of eating, as long as it's well balanced to ensure that you're getting the right mix of nutrients. Since veganism eliminates all animal-derived foods, it can be a bit of a challenge to meet your daily needs for certain nutrients that are primarily found in animal products, such as vitamin B12, vitamin D, calcium, iron, iodine, omega-3 fatty acids, zinc, and even protein.

Eat Your Veggies (and Fruits)

Every good diet starts with eating the recommended five or more servings of fruits and vegetables each day. This ensures that you get a wide range of vitamins, minerals, and antioxidants. These are the ingredients of a healthy diet and the nutrients that decrease your risk of diseases like heart disease, stroke, and many types of cancer. Of course, if your diet is solely plant-based, this part is a piece of cake (vegan cake, of course)!

Calcium

Calcium, which is crucial for building and maintaining strong bones and healthy muscles and nerves, is most commonly derived from animal products such as milk and other dairy products, but dark and leafy green vegetables—think kale, chard, collard greens, and broccoli—can provide sufficient quantities of calcium if you eat enough of them. You can also buy calcium-fortified juices, breads, cereals, soy milk, and other products to make sure you're getting enough. Most adults should consume 1,000 to 1,200 milligrams per day of calcium, either through food sources or as supplements.

Iodine

Iodine is another important nutrient that keeps your thyroid running smoothly. While many food sources of iodine are animal-based (dairy products, eggs, and fish), high concentrations can also be found in sea vegetables and strawberries. Iodized salt is fortified with iodine. Most adults need about 150 micrograms of iodine per day.

Iron

Iron is essential for developing red blood cells. Iron from meat is the most easily absorbed by the human body, but there are many plant-based sources of iron as well. Dried beans, iron-fortified cereals and breads, whole-grain foods, dark and leafy green vegetables, and dried fruit all contain ample amounts of iron. To maximize your absorption of the iron in these foods, combine them with rich sources of vitamin C, such as strawberries, citrus fruits, tomatoes, cabbage, and broccoli.

Omega-3 Fatty Acids

Omega-3 fatty acids help regulate metabolism and reduce the risk of cardiovascular disease. The most common dietary sources of these essential fatty acids are fish and eggs, but they can be found in canola oil or soy oil, walnuts, flaxseed, and soybeans.

Vitamin B12

Vitamin B12 is vitally important because it plays a key role in cell metabolism, the normal functioning of the brain and nervous system, and the formation of blood. It's found naturally in animal-based foods, including meat, fish, poultry, eggs, and dairy products, but many vegan-friendly foods are fortified with a synthetic form of vitamin B12, including soy milk and breakfast cereals. Supplements are also available in the form of pills, sublinguals, or injections. Aim to eat at least 3 micrograms per day in fortified foods or take a 10-microgram supplement daily.

Vitamin D

Like calcium, vitamin D is important for maintaining healthy bones. Many nondairy milks, however, are also fortified with vitamin D, as are many cereals and breads. Most adults need a minimum of 200 to 400 international units of vitamin D each day.

Zinc

Zinc plays a critical role in keeping the immune system strong as well as in cell division and the formation of proteins. Like iron, zinc from plant sources is not absorbed by the body as easily as that from animal products such as dairy. Good vegan sources of zinc include soybeans and products made with soybeans (such as tofu), whole grains, legumes, nuts, and wheat germ.

What to Eat

In the simplest terms, sticking to a vegan diet means eating only plant-based foods. So what does that mean in practice? It means you can eat cooked and raw vegetables and fruits, grains, vegetable oils, legumes (beans, peas, lentils, peanuts), nuts and nut butters, seeds and seed butters, cereals, eggless noodles and pasta, and baked goods such as breads, cookies, and cakes (so long as they are made without animal products). Here are just some of the foods available to you on a vegan diet:

Vegetables: asparagus, beets, broccoli, Brussels sprouts, cauliflower, chard, corn, cucumbers, eggplant, kale, lettuce, olives, onions, parsnips, potatoes, radishes, squash, sweet potatoes/yams, tomatoes, turnips

Fruits: apples, bananas, blackberries, blueberries, cherries, coconuts, grapes, mangos, melons, nectarines, papayas, peaches, pineapples, plums, raspberries, strawberries

Grains: amaranth, barley, farro, oats, quinoa, rice, wheat, and other grains; grain-based foods such as baked goods, breads, couscous, noodles (eggless)

Legumes: beans, lentils, peanuts and peanut butter, peas, soy products (tofu, miso, soy sauce, etc.)

THE IMPORTANCE OF PROTEIN

Protein, which is made up of essential amino acids, is an important nutrient for cell growth and repair and is one of the body's vital sources of energy. Typically, the average adult needs about 46 (women) to 56 (men) grams of protein per day, and vegans have to get it from plant sources. Fortunately, protein is easily found in the plant world, including in nuts, seeds, legumes, grains, and green vegetables.

Beans and legumes: Beans, peas, lentils, tofu, and peanuts are some of the best sources of protein for vegans, offering around 20 grams of protein per serving, which is about as much as a 3-ounce serving of meat. Four-Bean Chili (page 81), Curried Lentils (page 94), or Spicy Picnic Beans (page 95) will all provide a meal-size dose of protein. A handful of dry-roasted peanuts will give you a satisfying protein boost between meals.

Nuts and nut butters: Almonds, cashews, pecans, pistachios, and walnuts contain healthy fats in addition to about 5 grams of protein per ounce. Sprinkle some pecans on your breakfast of Apple and Cinnamon Oatmeal (page 31) or snack on Spiced Nuts (page 45).

Seeds and seed butters: Sesame, sunflower, hemp, chia, flax, poppy, and pumpkin seeds are all loaded with protein. Sunflower seeds contain more than 7 grams of protein in each ¼ cup serving. Snack on Wasabi-Toasted Pumpkin Seeds (page 46) or sprinkle a handful of sunflower seeds on your salad at lunch.

Whole grains: Whole wheat, brown rice, and barley provide 3 to 4 grams of protein per serving. Quinoa packs 8 grams of complete protein in a 1-cup serving. Get your day off to a good start with a breakfast of Warm Maple and Cinnamon Quinoa (page 30).

Green vegetables: A cup of chopped broccoli delivers 8 grams of protein, not to mention a nice boost of vitamins, antioxidants, and fiber. Sweet and Spicy Brussels Sprout Hash (page 104), Lemon Broccoli Rabe (page 109), or Green Beans Gremolata (page 102) served alongside a whole-grain side dish will make for a good protein-rich meal.

Nondairy milks: almond milk, cashew milk, coconut cream, coconut milk, hemp milk, rice milk, soy milk

Nuts and nut butters: almonds, almond butter, cashews, cashew butter, hazelnuts, hazelnut butter, pecans, walnuts

Oils: avocado, canola, coconut, flaxseed, grapeseed, olive, sesame

Seeds and seed butters: chia seeds, flaxseed, pine nuts, pumpkin seeds (pepitas), sesame seeds, tahini (sesame seed paste)

Sweeteners: agave nectar, fruit, maple syrup, stevia, sugar (some sugars use animal products, so make sure you buy vegan sugar)

Vegan substitutes: coconut butter, meatless deli slices, soy- or wheat gluten–based faux meat products such as tofu hot dogs, vegan cheese made from either nuts or tapioca, vegan egg replacer, vegan margarine, vegan mayonnaise, veggie burgers

What Not to Eat

Transitioning to a vegan diet will likely mean you'll need to revisit your standard foods for every meal, even if you were already an ovo-lacto vegetarian.

Here are some foods that you will want to replace in your diet with vegan options:

Dairy products: Milk, cheese, butter, ghee, and foods made with dairy products, including pastry crust, yogurt, ice cream, and so on; whey and casein, ingredients that come from milk, are common in many foods, including margarine, many boxed cereals and cereal bars, breads and bread crumbs, crackers, and even some soy- and grain-based cheese substitutes

Eggs: Any type of eggs, whether from chickens, ducks, ostriches, salmon, or other animals, as well as foods made with eggs, such as mayonnaise, noodles, pancakes, waffles, cakes, cookies, and many other baked goods

Honey: Bees make honey, rendering it a no-no for the vegan diet. Watch out for honey in many healthy brands of cereal, whole-grain breads, cookies and other baked goods, and beverages

Meat, poultry, and seafood: Chicken, fish, beef, pork, lamb, veal, shellfish, and so on, as well as foods made with meat or meat by-products, such as lard, marrow, and suet

Twelve Surprising Nonvegan Foods

A vegan diet requires that you refrain from eating animal by-products. Many of these foods are obvious, but there are some nonvegan ingredients hidden in items you'd never think were off-limits.

WHAT ABOUT ALLERGIES?

Steering clear of common food allergens like gluten, soy, or nuts is where your newly honed label-reading skills will come in particularly handy.

Gluten-Free

Following a diet that is both gluten-free and vegan poses a particular challenge in that many of the grain-based protein sources available to vegans contain gluten. Seitan, for instance, is a common meat substitute that is made of wheat gluten. There are, however, numerous gluten-free, high-protein grains that can be substituted for wheat, barley, rye, and spelt, such as amaranth, quinoa, and rice. Other gluten-free and vegan protein sources include soy (edamame, tofu, and some meat substitutes), legumes (beans, lentils, peanuts, and the like), nuts, seeds, and green vegetables.

Breads, cereals, and pastas made with wheat are obviously no-nos, but look for gluten-free noodles and breads made with alternative flours like rice, sorghum, almond, or hazelnut.

Watch out for gluten in soy sauce, malt vinegar, and other seasonings as well. A great substitute for soy sauce is a sauce made of either soy-based or coconut-based aminos. Look for it at any health food store.

Soy-Free

Vegans who are allergic to soy face a similar issue to those sensitive to gluten in that many vegan meat and dairy substitutes are made of soy—soy milk, soy cheese, tofu, tofu dogs, tofu burgers, and so on. Luckily, there are lots of soy-free vegan foods available.

Instead of soy milk, you can choose from rice milk, hemp milk, almond milk, cashew milk, or coconut milk. Dairy-free cheeses can be made with nuts or even tapioca. These days there are even soy-free meat substitutes on the market, and coconut aminos make a great alternative to soy sauce.

Nut-Free

A tree nut and/or peanut allergy is easier to accommodate on a vegan diet than either a gluten or soy allergy since nuts are not quite as ubiquitous in meat substitutes, but you do still have to be careful and read labels.

As far as substitutions go, seeds add similar crunch to salads and baked goods, and seed butters can often be substituted for nut butters and seed oils for nut oils in recipes. Try sunflower, sesame, pumpkin, chia seeds, and flaxseed in recipes, as snacks, or as butters. They'll provide the heart-healthy fat you need, and you'll hardly miss the nuts.

It's essential to do your research and read labels carefully—even those labels for products you'd never suspect of harboring foods derived from animals.

Following is a list of foods that may contain animal products. In all likelihood; at least a few of these will come as a surprise.

1. **Refried beans:** Refried beans are often made with lard. When buying canned beans, you can likely rely on a "vegetarian" label to avoid this ingredient, but be sure to ask in a restaurant before digging into those *frijoles*.

2. **Orange juice:** The most common source of omega-3s is fish, which means that any food or beverage that is fortified with omega-3s is suspect, including that glass of heart-healthy orange juice accompanying your breakfast. The same goes for omega-3 supplements in pill form. To ensure you get enough of this important nutrient, it's probably safest to stick with plant-based food sources such as flaxseed, chia seeds, or purslane.

3. **Candy:** Gelatin is made from the skin, bones, and hooves of pigs and cows. Foods that contain gelatin include gummy bears, marshmallows, Altoids, and many other candies. Additional foods that often have gelatin include Jell-O, pudding, many jams, and even some smoothies and packaged nuts.

4. **Worcestershire sauce:** This common sauce is almost always flavored with anchovies, though vegetarian versions are available.

5. **Some breads:** Really—some bagels contain an amino acid, L-cysteine, which is derived from human hair or poultry feathers!

6. **Cakes and cake mixes:** Some cake brands contain beef fat, of all things.

7. **Beer and wine:** Many alcoholic beverages use isinglass (fish bladders), gelatin, or egg whites in the clarifying process. These substances won't be listed on the ingredients list, so it could take some serious digging to find brands that are strictly free of animal products.

8. **Red food coloring:** Certain foods contain a red dye that comes from the scales of the cochineal beetle. This may be listed in the ingredients as Red Dye #4 or Natural Red #4.

9. **Flavored potato chips:** Some have dairy or animal fat. Who knew?

10. **Nondairy creamers:** It's true. Many are made with caseinate, which is derived from milk.

11. **Margarine:** This is another food that's sold as a dairy alternative but often contains whey or casein, both of which come from milk. It also might have gelatin or animal fat (suet).

12. **Soy- or grain-based cheese alternatives:** Shockingly, though they are sold as dairy alternatives, these foods sometimes contain dairy in the form of casein or whey.

How to Get Started

Becoming a vegan is more than a matter of tweaking your day-to-day menu—it's a major lifestyle change and a substantial undertaking, even if you're already a vegetarian. Making the decision to live an animal product–free life is only the first step. Being clear about your reasons for making this change will help guide you and keep you true to your goals when the going gets tough.

Begin Slowly

Once you've made the choice to cut out animal products, you may be tempted to dive in headfirst, but eliminating one food group at a time will make the transition easier and you'll be more likely to maintain the change over time. It may seem counterintuitive, but start by eliminating the foods with animal by-products that are least central to your daily diet—like marshmallows and Worcestershire sauce. Go through your kitchen cabinets, read labels, and toss (or give away) anything that contains sneaky animal products like gelatin, casein, Red Dye #4, whey, or animal fat. Once you've done all that, you'll have some success under your belt and a base of confidence. Next, tackle a bigger food group like eggs or dairy. Give yourself some time to adjust to life without each of these food groups before moving on to the next.

Another way to ease into a vegan lifestyle is to stick to vegan eating only when you're at home, where you're able to control what you eat more easily. Do this for a period of time before extending it to meals that are away from home.

Study Up

In addition to researching what animal products might be hiding in your food under unsuspicious-sounding names, take a bit of time to learn about the nutrients your body needs, paying particular attention to those that normally come primarily from animal products—calcium, iron, iodine, and so on (see previous list of vitamins, minerals, and antioxidants). Familiarize yourself with vegan sources of these nutrients where possible, or visit your local health food store and ask about supplements.

Look at Your New Diet as an Adventure

Some people get anxious about all the new rules that come along with a vegan diet, but if you view it as an adventure, you can relax and enjoy exploring new cuisines and discovering new foods. Give yourself time to browse at the market, delight in finding new staples to replace your nonvegan standards, and uncover some delicious foods you never knew existed. Let yourself experiment in the kitchen, too. Learn to cook amazing vegan dishes (the recipes in this book are a great place to start).

Scout Out the Neighborhood

If you're lucky, there's a vegan restaurant and a health food store or two where you live, but even if there isn't, don't fret. No matter where you are, there's likely a good source for plenty of vegan food. Any decent supermarket these days carries milk substitutes (soy, almond, rice, etc.), tofu, veggie burgers, and faux meats. Health and natural food stores like Whole Foods, Sprouts, and Trader Joe's offer even more vegan-friendly options. Farmers' markets are great places to buy local, organic, and seasonal fruits and vegetables. Many also have stands offering artisan baked goods and ready-to-eat meals that may be vegan-friendly.

Gear Up

You really don't need to invest in any special cooking equipment in order to make vegan food, but slow cookers and pressure cookers are great for cooking dried beans and other vegan foods. A rice cooker also comes in handy.

Seven-Day Meal Plan

Having a detailed plan is a great way to get you started on the right track. It's like a road map that shows you exactly where to turn every step of the way.

This seven-day meal plan is designed to start you on the right foot by providing a guideline for you to follow for the first week of your vegan diet. Once you've been immersed in the vegan lifestyle for as little as a week or two, you'll likely find that choosing vegan foods becomes second nature.

The meal plan includes a number of the recipes from this book. These recipes, of course, are all easy to make, full of flavor, and free of animal products of any kind.

Day One
Breakfast: Warm Maple and Cinnamon Quinoa*
Lunch: Kale and Root Vegetable Salad*
Dinner: Portuguese Black Beans and Rice*

Day Two
Breakfast: Breakfast Parfaits*
Lunch: Brown Rice and Pepper Salad*
Dinner: Grilled Pesto Tofu* with Spicy Swiss Chard* and eggless pasta

Day Three
Breakfast: Green Breakfast Smoothie*
Lunch: Tempeh Reuben Sandwich*
Dinner: Easy Corn Chowder* with Green Beans Gremolata*

Day Four
Breakfast: Sweet Potato and Kale Hash*
Lunch: Avocado and Spicy Sprout Sandwich*
Dinner: Black Bean Soup* with green salad

Day Five
Breakfast: Apple and Cinnamon Oatmeal*
Lunch: Grilled Cannellini Bean, Spinach, and Artichoke Panini*
Dinner: Fried Rice* with Orange and Soy Tofu*

Day Six
Breakfast: Blueberry and Chia Smoothie*
Lunch: Seitan Barbecue Sandwich*
Dinner: Curried Lentils* with brown rice

Day Seven
Breakfast: Orange French Toast*
Lunch: Pear and Arugula Salad*
Dinner: Four-Bean Chili*

Ten Tips for a Happy Vegan Life

Becoming a vegan isn't an easy choice, and frankly, many people aren't able to stick it out. The list of reasons people give for reverting to their old animal product–eating ways is long. Some develop nutrient deficiencies and resulting health problems, while others have difficulty focusing or become depressed (likely also due to nutrient deficiencies), and still others struggle with unsupportive families or friends or the difficulty of being the only vegan in town. Here are ten tips that can help you avoid these downfalls and more.

1. **Take supplements that help fight depression:** Since deficiencies in nutrients like vitamin B12, vitamin D, iodine, and iron can all contribute to existing depression or even bring it on, supplementing these nutrients from the get-go can make all the difference.

2. **Exercise regularly:** Exercise is important for everyone, but when you alter your diet it can be especially helpful in keeping you feeling good and fighting fatigue. Plus, when you're physically fit, you are more inclined to want to put only healthy foods into your body.

3. **Eat protein:** As discussed earlier, there is really no reason that vegans should have trouble meeting their protein requirements, but it's a good idea to make sure you're eating at least two servings of protein-rich foods like beans, nuts, and seeds each day.

4. **Eat fat:** Your body needs fat in order to absorb many vitamins and nutrients, so eating a diet that is too low in fat is detrimental. Cutting out high-fat foods like meat and dairy products can leave you feeling hungry, tired, and unwell. Choose healthy vegan sources of fat like nuts, seeds, nut and seed oils, coconut, olives, and avocados.

5. **Pile on the flavor:** By cutting animal products out of your diet, you automatically eliminate a huge source of fat. And let's face it—fat makes food taste good. As previously mentioned, there are plenty of delicious vegan sources of fat, but don't forget about other ways to add flavor. Spices, fresh herbs, sun-dried tomatoes, dried fruits, and assorted salts add intense flavor.

6. **Create new favorites:** Rather than trying to enjoy your favorite meat- or dairy-containing dishes by simply cutting out the offending ingredients, which will likely only leave you disappointed, try creating new versions of your favorites using vegan-substitute ingredients. Dairy-free cheese pizza with caramelized vegetables may just be delicious enough to make you forget all about that *quattro formaggio* version you once adored.

7. **Cook in batches:** Make large batches of rice, beans, and your favorite vegan soups and stews, and store individual portions in your fridge or freezer. Having ready-to-eat meals on hand can take a lot of the stress out of any restrictive way of eating. You can stop slaving over cooking each and every meal, freeing yourself to explore new ingredients or cooking techniques when you have the time.

8. **Pay attention to cravings:** When your body craves certain foods, it's often a sign that you're lacking a particular nutrient like calcium or vitamin B12, for example.

Since certain nutrients do come primarily from animal products, you may find yourself craving meat, but you can find vegan ways to supplement those nutrients and banish those cravings.

9. **Stock up on vegan snacks:** One of the biggest challenges of any restrictive diet is that moment when you're away from home, starving, and need a quick bite to eat, but there are no appropriate options available. In such an instance, your choices are to go hungry or cave in and choose something with off-limits ingredients. You'll avoid this situation altogether if you stash vegan snacks in your car, your desk drawer at work, your pockets, and your purse or backpack. Single-serving packs of nuts or seeds, trail mix, dried fruits, roasted chickpeas, or dairy-free cereal or protein bars are good choices that don't need refrigeration and can be eaten on the go.

10. **Find support:** One of the things many people fail to think about before launching a vegan lifestyle is the emotional aspect. The social implications can be huge, especially if you don't have many friends who are vegan. It can be lonely being the only vegan in town. Whether you find support in your social circle or with strangers online, having someone you can talk to about your day-to-day challenges and swap recipes and food tips with can mean the difference between success and failure.

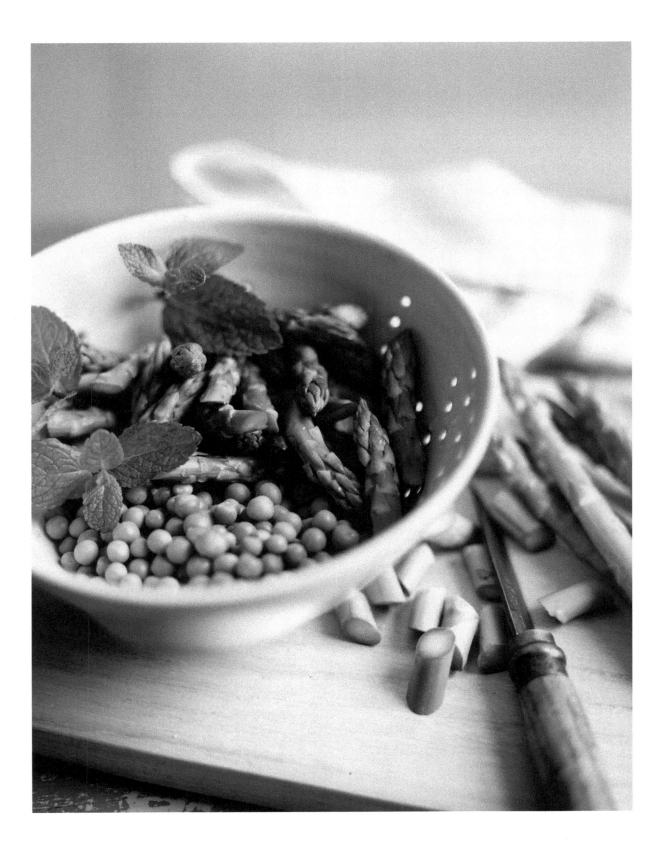

2

Saving Time and Money

Plan Meals in Advance

One of the best ways to save money at the grocery store is to sit down each weekend and plan your meals for the week. Make a list of what you will serve each day. When planning your meals, check your refrigerator for any perishables you need to consume soon and incorporate them into your recipes.

To save more time, you can double some dinner recipes to use for lunch or leftovers later in the week.

Make a Shopping List

If you use a shopping list every time you go to the store, you'll be far more likely to avoid making impulse buys, which can save money. Before making your shopping list, be sure you also check the pantry to see what you may need to replenish. Then, using your meal plan, make a shopping list of the ingredients you need.

You can further increase your savings by shopping according to store specials. Many grocery stores now have saving cards with tablet, smartphone, or computer applications that allow you to view real-time store circulars and download coupons to your device. If you prefer a lower-tech option, you can also clip coupons and use store ads that come in the mail or newspaper. Using these tools as you plan meals is an excellent way to save money.

What to Shop For

Setting up your vegan pantry is fairly straightforward. Every ingredient should be nutrient-dense. Packaged foods such as cereals, orange juice, and vegan milks can boost your intake of nutrients since they are fortified with important vitamins and minerals.

Many of these ingredients are available in bulk at your local supermarket, so you may want to invest in a few airtight containers to store unpackaged or loosely packaged foods. It's also a good idea to start a collection bin for food scraps, because almost all vegetable peelings and excess cuttings can be used to make vegetable stock.

Vacuum-sealed packages of vegan milk are becoming widely available. Vegan sour cream, usually derived from soy, is similar in texture and taste to cow milk sour cream.

For the Pantry

JARS, BOXES, AND CANS

- Canned pumpkin
- Jarred chopped ginger
- Soy sauce
- Coconut oil
- Unsweetened coconut milk
- Unsweetened almond milk
- Unsweetened soy milk
- Jarred roasted red peppers
- Dried mushrooms, especially porcini
- Salsa
- Pickled jalapeños
- Jarred artichoke hearts
- Jarred sauerkraut
- Dill pickles
- Barbecue sauce
- Egg-free mayonnaise
- Boxed vegetable stock
- Chili paste, Sriracha or sambal, chipotle chili paste
- Peanut butter
- Nutritional yeast
- Cornstarch
- Tamarind paste
- Tomato sauce
- Pitted dates

PRODUCE

- Garlic
- Yellow onions
- Shallots
- Canned tomatoes (a variety of crushed, diced, and whole)
- Sweet potatoes
- Waxy potatoes such as Yukon Gold
- Olives
- Rutabaga
- Parsnips
- Jicama

GRAINS, NUTS, SEEDS, AND LEGUMES

- Chia seeds
- Almonds
- Brazil nuts
- Peanuts
- Pecans
- Pumpkin seeds
- Sunflower seeds
- Walnuts
- Pine nuts
- Sesame seeds
- Couscous
- Lentils
- Whole-wheat flour
- Long-grain brown and white rice
- Oats
- Quinoa
- Unsweetened cereals
- Whole-grain bread
- Whole-grain crackers
- Soba noodles
- Bean thread (also called cellophane) noodles or other rice noodles
- Whole-grain pita
- Whole-wheat spaghetti
- Rice noodles
- Wild rice
- Black beans
- Chickpeas (also called garbanzo beans)
- Kidney beans
- Pinto beans
- Cannellini, navy, or other white beans

OIL AND VINEGAR

- Olive oil
- Sesame oil
- Balsamic vinegar
- Apple cider vinegar
- Unseasoned rice vinegar

SWEETENERS AND FLAVORINGS

- Cocoa powder
- Maple syrup
- Agave syrup
- Dijon mustard
- Pomegranate juice

For the Refrigerator

Fresh fruits and vegetables are central to a vegan lifestyle, and eating them in a wide range of colors will add excitement and nutrients to your diet. Proteins such as seitan and tempeh can last for quite a while if their packages are unopened and they're easy to freeze. Firm tofu does not have a long shelf life once it's been opened, and it does not freeze well, so purchase only as much as you need for a given recipe.

- Hass avocados
- Lemons and limes
- Spinach
- Kale
- Arugula
- Lettuces
- Tomatoes
- Cucumbers
- Fresh herbs—cilantro, parsley, tarragon, basil, and mint
- Apples
- Fresh alliums such as scallions and chives
- Radishes
- Mushrooms
- Hummus
- Tahini (puréed sesame seeds)
- Tempeh
- Sliced seitan
- Carrots
- Celery
- Eggplant
- Bell peppers
- Fennel
- Leeks
- Green beans
- Peas and snap peas
- Brussels sprouts
- Broccoli and broccoli rabe
- Swiss chard
- Cauliflower
- Bean sprouts
- Red and green cabbage
- Zucchini
- Extra-firm tofu
- Vegan sour cream
- Vegan cheeses
- Vegan creamer

For the Freezer

Most people underuse their freezer, but it can add value and variety to your cooking routine. Fruits and vegetables can be prepared in season, when they are least expensive, then frozen for later use. You can freeze leftovers in portion sizes and enjoy them later as a grab-n-go lunch.

- Fruits—berries, peaches, and mangos
- Concentrated apple juice
- Concentrated orange juice
- Spinach
- Corn
- Peas
- Bags of precut mixed vegetables
- Vegan ice cream

For the Spice Rack

Variety is the spice of life. Just a few spices, purchased in small amounts to ensure freshness, can make a huge difference in the flavor of your food. Purchase whole, unprocessed spices and grind them yourself just before you cook to ensure maximum flavor.

- Black peppercorns
- California and Turkish bay leaves
- Cinnamon
- Nutmeg
- Allspice
- Thyme
- Cumin
- Five-spice powder
- Wasabi powder
- Sea salt
- Cayenne pepper
- Chipotle powder
- Red pepper flakes
- Rosemary
- Curry powder
- Italian seasoning
- Star anise
- Smoked sweet paprika
- Garlic powder
- Cajun seasoning
- Coriander
- Garam masala
- Jerk seasoning

Use Prepared Ingredients

Another way to save time is to use prepared ingredients. These ingredients differ from processed foods. Prepared, nonprocessed ingredients are still whole foods that haven't been manipulated or are minimally manipulated. Processed foods, on the other hand, contain unnatural ingredients, such as artificial flavors, preservatives, and dyes. For example, frozen corn is a prepared food, while a frozen corn enchilada is a processed food.

Healthy Prepared Substitutes for Fresh Foods

You can substitute the following prepared foods for fresh foods in your recipes. When doing so, check the ingredients on the package to ensure you are choosing products that minimize artificial ingredients.

- Canned beans and legumes
- Canned coconut milk
- Canned fruits that are not stored in syrup
- Canned tomatoes
- Canned vegetables, such as pumpkin, squash, and green beans
- Dried fruits
- Dried mushrooms
- Frozen fruit and berries without added sugar
- Frozen or chopped onions
- Frozen prepared grains, such as rice or quinoa
- Frozen vegetables
- Nut butters
- Nut milks, such as almond and coconut milk
- Prepared guacamole
- Prepared salsa
- Roasted nuts and seeds
- Unsweetened lemon and lime juice
- Vegetable stock or broth

Reduce Waste

When you're planning meals, minimizing the amount of food you throw away can help you save money. Some waste-reduction methods include:

- Sticking to your shopping list.
- Saving vegetable trimmings—such as mushroom stems, onion tops, carrot peels, celery leaves, leek trimmings, and herb stems to make vegetable stock.
- Knowing how to store foods properly (see pages 22–23).
- Keeping your refrigerator and cupboards organized so you always know what you have.
- Reusing or freezing leftovers.
- Labeling all stored items in the freezer with ingredients and the date you froze them. Rotating the stock to use the oldest first.
- Purchasing reusable containers for refrigerating or freezing.
- Sanitizing bottles or jars in your dishwasher and using them to store leftovers.
- Setting your refrigerator and freezer temperatures appropriately. Set the refrigerator at or below 40°F and freezer at or below 0°F.
- Composting food scraps.

4 WAYS TO CUT TOFU

You don't need an advanced degree in butchery to know how to break down a block of tofu, but learning the best way to get a variety of shapes and sizes of tofu pieces will go a long way in your vegan cookery.

Cubes

Cubes are probably the most common shape you'll see in recipes. They work for saucy dishes where you want each mouthful to be coated in the flavorful sauce, and for soups or stews where it's helpful to have bite-size pieces that can easily be picked up with a spoon.

To cut cubes, start by making three evenly spaced vertical slices down the length of the block, which will give you three equal-sized slabs. Keeping the slabs together in block form, turn the whole thing on its side and make three more vertical slices (these will be perpendicular to the first three slices). Now you have nine sticks. Next, cut four vertical slices perpendicular to the last three slices you made. Voilà—twenty-seven bite-size cubes of tofu.

Small Triangles

Once you've sliced your tofu slab into cubes (see instructions), you can turn them into small triangles by slicing each cube in half on the diagonal.

Slabs

Slabs are best for grilling, broiling, or searing. To make them, set your block of tofu in front of you on the cutting board with the long side toward you. Cut this right down the middle so that you have two halves on the left and right. Next, cut each half in half so that you have quarters. Now cut those quarters in half. Bingo—eight slabs of tofu ready for the grill.

Large Triangles

These can be grilled, broiled, or seared and are a bit smaller than full slabs, making them great for appetizers or salads. They're also ideal for deep-frying and dipping into sauce.

To cut large triangles, follow the instructions for cutting slabs, then lay each slab flat on the cutting board and cut it in half diagonally.

Proper Storage Methods

Vegetable Stock

- Store in an airtight container and refrigerate if you plan to use it within the week.
- Store in an airtight container and freeze for up to 12 months.
- Freeze in an ice-cube tray and then transfer ice cubes to an airtight container for up to 12 months. Use the cubes when you need a small amount of stock.

Dried Legumes and Grains

- Store in an airtight container at room temperature indefinitely.

Nuts and Seeds

- Store raw nuts and seeds in a tightly sealed container at room temperature for up to 3 months, in the refrigerator for up to 6 months, or in the freezer for 1 year.
- Roasted nuts can be stored in a tightly sealed container at room temperature for up to 1 year, or in the refrigerator for up to 2 years.

Herbs and Spices

- Store fresh herbs you plan to use within a week with their stems in a glass of water in the refrigerator.
- Freeze fresh herbs in olive oil in an ice-cube tray and then transfer to a tightly sealed container for up to 1 year. Use 1 tablespoon chopped fresh herbs per cube.
- Store whole dried spices in tightly sealed containers for 2 to 3 years.
- Store ground spices in tightly sealed containers for 6 months to 1 year.
- Store dried leafy herbs in tightly sealed containers for 3 to 6 months.

Potatoes, Onions, and Garlic

Fresh potatoes, onions, shallots, and garlic can be stored in the refrigerator crisper drawer for up to a week. Potatoes, onions, garlic, and shallots (those with a papery or dry skin) should be stored in a breathable container, such as an open-top paper bag or a basket in a cool, dark place for 2 to 3 months. If you plan to eat the potatoes or onions sooner, you can store them on the counter in a breathable bowl, such as a colander, for about 4 weeks.

Nut Butter

- Store in original packaging tightly sealed in the refrigerator for up to 1 year.

Leafy Greens

- As soon as you purchase the greens, remove any damaged leaves.
- Rinse the leaves in cold water to remove any dirt.
- Dry the leaves thoroughly, first in a colander or salad spinner, and then by blotting any excess water.
- Roll the greens loosely in a dry paper towel.
- Place in an unsealed plastic bag in the refrigerator's crisper drawer for up to 1 week.

Other Fresh Fruits and Vegetables

Store in the refrigerator's crisper for up to 2 weeks. You can also cut leftover fruits or vegetables into chunks and freeze them in a tightly sealed container for up to 1 year.

Tofu

Store tofu in a tightly sealed container or original packaging in the refrigerator. Open tofu needs to be consumed within 1 week. You can also cut leftover tofu into chunks and freeze on a tray on parchment paper. Once the chunks freeze, transfer them to a tightly sealed container and keep frozen for up to 1 year.

Prepare Foods ahead of Time

You can save time by preparing foods before you need to use them in recipes. Many foods can be prepped when you have time and then stored for later use. Prepare ingredients on the weekend or on your days off, and then either refrigerate or freeze in a tightly sealed container until you are ready to use them. For example, if you use bulk items, such as grains or legumes, prep them on your days off and they'll be ready to use in recipes.

Common Ingredients That Can Be Prepped ahead of Time

You can prepare the following foods ahead of time and store, tightly sealed, in the refrigerator for up to 1 week or in the freezer for up to 6 months:

- Chopped vegetables
- Dried legumes, such as lentils, chickpeas, split peas, and beans
- Grains, such as rice and quinoa
- Marinades
- Salads (without dressing)
- Sauces, such as tomato sauce or salsa
- Soups and stews
- Vegetable stock
- Vinaigrettes

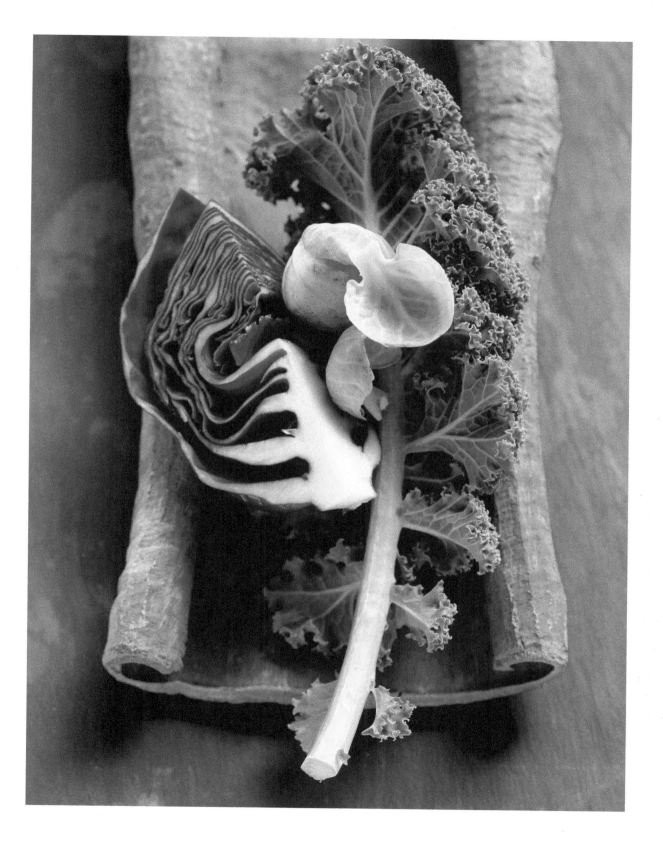

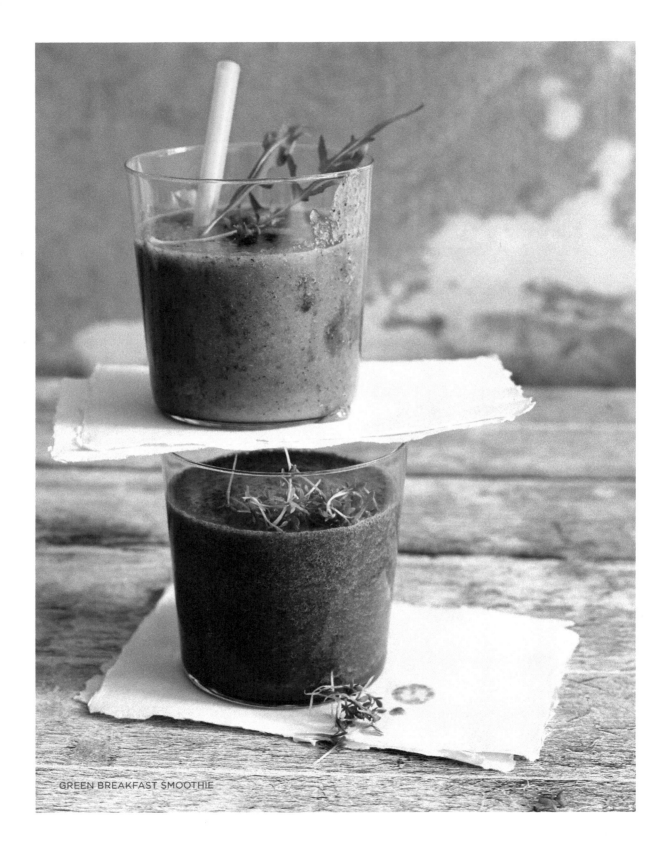

GREEN BREAKFAST SMOOTHIE

3

Breakfasts

SERVES 2

PREP TIME
10 MINUTES

COOKING TIME
0 MINUTES

Green Breakfast Smoothie

This smoothie is a great way to add leafy greens to your diet. Thickened with flavorful banana and sweetened with juicy oranges and berries, you'll hardly even notice the savory flavor of the spinach, but the bright green color will give you confidence that you're drinking plenty of health-giving, plant-based nutrients.

Tip Drinking your smoothie immediately after you make it ensures that you'll get the maximum nutrition from the ingredients. If you're short on time, put it in a travel mug to sip on your commute.

½ BANANA, SLICED

2 CUPS SPINACH OR OTHER GREENS,
   SUCH AS KALE

1 CUP SLICED BERRIES OF YOUR
   CHOOSING, FRESH OR FROZEN

1 ORANGE, PEELED AND CUT INTO
   SEGMENTS

1 CUP UNSWEETENED NONDAIRY MILK

1 CUP ICE

1. In a blender, combine all the ingredients.

2. Starting with the blender on low speed, begin blending the smoothie, gradually increasing blender speed until smooth. Serve immediately.

Blueberry and Chia Smoothie

Chia seeds are one of the best plant-based sources of omega-3 fatty acids. Blueberries and cocoa powder are both nutrition powerhouses, too, loading this quick breakfast with vitamins, minerals, and antioxidants.

Tip Chia seeds contribute protein and other nutrients to this healthy smoothie, but they are also what give it its satisfyingly thick consistency. Soaking chia seeds in liquid for 5 to 10 minutes creates a dense gel that adds body. This method can also be used to make puddings.

2 TABLESPOONS CHIA SEEDS

2 CUPS UNSWEETENED
   NONDAIRY MILK

2 CUPS BLUEBERRIES, FRESH
   OR FROZEN

2 TABLESPOONS PURE MAPLE SYRUP
   OR AGAVE

2 TABLESPOONS COCOA POWDER

1. Soak the chia seeds in the almond milk for 5 minutes.

2. In a blender, combine the soaked chia seeds, almond milk, blueberries, maple syrup, and cocoa powder and blend until smooth. Serve immediately.

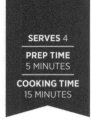
Warm Maple and Cinnamon Quinoa

High in protein and quick to make, quinoa is a great alternative to traditional hot breakfast cereals like oatmeal or cream of wheat. This version is fragrant with maple syrup and cinnamon, making it a hearty and satisfying meal that's perfect on a cold morning.

Tip Quinoa cooks fast, but on busy mornings you may not even have 15 minutes to spare. Make a batch ahead of time and reheat it in the microwave for an almost-instant breakfast. Stir in the nuts or seeds just before serving.

1 CUP UNSWEETENED NONDAIRY MILK

1 CUP WATER

1 CUP QUINOA, RINSED

1 TEASPOON CINNAMON

¼ CUP CHOPPED PECANS OR OTHER NUTS OR SEEDS, SUCH AS CHIA, SUNFLOWER SEEDS, OR ALMONDS

2 TABLESPOONS PURE MAPLE SYRUP OR AGAVE

1. In a medium saucepan over medium-high heat, bring the almond milk, water, and quinoa to a boil. Lower the heat to medium-low and cover. Simmer until the liquid is mostly absorbed and the quinoa softens, about 15 minutes.

2. Turn off the heat and allow to sit, covered, for 5 minutes. Stir in the cinnamon, pecans, and syrup. Serve hot.

Apple and Cinnamon Oatmeal

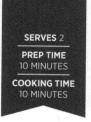
SERVES 2

PREP TIME
10 MINUTES

COOKING TIME
10 MINUTES

This classic hot breakfast cereal is a kid favorite because the oats are cooked in apple cider, giving them intense apple flavor and a boost of sweetness. If you like your oatmeal even sweeter, add the maple syrup or agave.

1¼ CUPS APPLE CIDER

1 APPLE, PEELED, CORED, AND CHOPPED

⅔ CUP ROLLED OATS

1 TEASPOON GROUND CINNAMON

1 TABLESPOON PURE MAPLE SYRUP OR AGAVE (OPTIONAL)

1. In a medium saucepan, bring the apple cider to a boil over medium-high heat. Stir in the apple, oats, and cinnamon.

2. Bring the cereal to a boil and turn down heat to low. Simmer until the oatmeal thickens, 3 to 4 minutes. Spoon into two bowls and sweeten with maple syrup, if using. Serve hot.

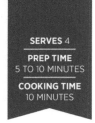
Spiced Orange Breakfast Couscous

Loaded with protein and fiber, quinoa makes a filling breakfast that will keep you going until lunch. This version—cooked in orange juice for bright, sweet flavor and combined with spices, dried fruits, and nuts—is especially satisfying.

3 CUPS ORANGE JUICE

1½ CUPS COUSCOUS

1 TEASPOON GROUND CINNAMON

¼ TEASPOON GROUND CLOVES

½ CUP DRIED FRUIT, SUCH AS RAISINS OR APRICOTS

½ CUP CHOPPED ALMONDS OR OTHER NUTS OR SEEDS

1. In a small saucepan, bring the orange juice to a boil. Add the couscous, cinnamon, and cloves and remove from heat. Cover the pan with a lid and allow to sit until the couscous softens, about 5 minutes.

2. Fluff the couscous with a fork and stir in the dried fruit and nuts. Serve immediately.

Broiled Grapefruit with Cinnamon Pitas

Half a grapefruit has been a favorite breakfast choice for generations. Drizzling the fruit with agave and caramelizing it under the broiler gives it a light sweetness that pairs perfectly with toasty cinnamon-sugar pita wedges.

2 WHOLE-WHEAT PITAS, CUT
   INTO WEDGES
2 TABLESPOONS COCONUT
   OIL, MELTED
1 TABLESPOON GROUND CINNAMON

2 TABLESPOONS BROWN SUGAR
1 GRAPEFRUIT, HALVED
2 TABLESPOONS PURE MAPLE SYRUP
   OR AGAVE

1. Preheat the oven to 375°F. Line a baking sheet with parchment paper.

2. Spread pita wedges in a single layer on a baking sheet and brush with melted coconut oil.

3. In a small bowl, combine the cinnamon and brown sugar and sprinkle over the pita wedges.

4. Bake in preheated oven until the wedges are crisp, about 8 minutes. Transfer the pita wedges to a plate and set aside.

5. Turn the oven to broil. Place the grapefruit halves on the baking sheet. Drizzle the maple syrup over the top of the grapefruit, if using. Broil until the syrup bubbles and begins to crystallize, 3 to 5 minutes. Serve immediately.

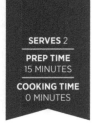

Breakfast Parfaits

The secret to these parfaits is thick, full-fat coconut milk, so don't substitute a light version. Layered with crunchy granola, protein-packed walnuts, and juicy berries, this healthy breakfast tastes more like a naughty dessert.

Tip Refrigerating the can of coconut milk overnight makes it easy to separate the thick coconut cream from the liquid coconut milk. Pour the milk off into a storage container and save it for another use (it's a great replacement for cream in your morning coffee).

ONE 14-OUNCE CAN COCONUT MILK,
    REFRIGERATED OVERNIGHT
1 CUP GRANOLA

½ CUP WALNUTS
1 CUP SLICED STRAWBERRIES OR
    OTHER SEASONAL BERRIES

1. Pour off the canned coconut-milk liquid and retain the solids.

2. In two parfait glasses, layer the coconut-milk solids, granola, walnuts, and strawberries. Serve immediately.

Orange French Toast

SERVES 4

PREP TIME
15 MINUTES

COOKING TIME
10 MINUTES

What could make for a better breakfast than thick slices of French bread soaked in a spiced custard thickened with bananas and flavored with orange juice and zest and then browned in coconut oil? The fruit in the custard makes this plenty sweet on its own, but go ahead and add a drizzle of maple syrup if you are so inclined.

3 VERY RIPE BANANAS

1 CUP UNSWEETENED
    NONDAIRY MILK

ZEST AND JUICE OF 1 ORANGE

1 TEASPOON GROUND CINNAMON

¼ TEASPOON GRATED NUTMEG

4 SLICES FRENCH BREAD

1 TABLESPOON COCONUT OIL

1. In a blender, combine the bananas, almond milk, orange juice and zest, cinnamon, and nutmeg and blend until smooth. Pour the mixture into a 9-by-13-inch baking dish. Soak the bread in the mixture for 5 minutes on each side.

2. While the bread soaks, heat a griddle or sauté pan over medium-high heat. Melt the coconut oil in the pan and swirl to coat. Cook the bread slices until golden brown on both sides, about 5 minutes each. Serve immediately.

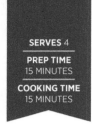

Pumpkin Pancakes

Baking powder and apple cider vinegar give these pancakes plenty of fluff, eliminating the need for eggs. Enriched with pumpkin purée and pumpkin pie spices, this healthy breakfast tastes more like a Thanksgiving dessert—not that anyone's complaining about that!

2 CUPS UNSWEETENED ALMOND MILK

1 TEASPOON APPLE CIDER
    VINEGAR

2½ CUPS WHOLE-WHEAT FLOUR

2 TABLESPOONS BAKING POWDER

½ TEASPOON BAKING SODA

1 TEASPOON SEA SALT

1 TEASPOON PUMPKIN PIE SPICE OR
    ½ TEASPOON GROUND CINNAMON
    PLUS ¼ TEASPOON GRATED
    NUTMEG PLUS ¼ TEASPOON
    GROUND ALLSPICE

½ CUP CANNED PUMPKIN PURÉE

1 CUP WATER

1 TABLESPOON COCONUT OIL

1. In a small bowl, combine the almond milk and apple cider vinegar. Set aside.

2. In a large bowl, whisk together the flour, baking powder, baking soda, salt, and pumpkin pie spice.

3. In another large bowl, combine the almond milk mixture, pumpkin purée, and water, whisking to mix well.

4. Add the wet ingredients to the dry ingredients and fold together until the dry ingredients are just moistened. You will still have a few streaks of flour in the bowl.

5. In a nonstick pan or griddle over medium-high heat, melt the coconut oil and swirl to coat. Pour the batter into the pan ¼ cup at a time and cook until the pancakes are browned, about 5 minutes per side. Serve immediately.

Sweet Potato and Kale Hash

SERVES 2

PREP TIME
10 MINUTES

COOKING TIME
15 MINUTES

Start your day with super-nutritious sweet potatoes, which are a great plant-based source of both the iron and vitamin D that those on a vegan diet need. Here they're panfried with herbs and other healthy veggies for a quick and satisfying savory breakfast.

Tip Sweet potatoes can take up to an hour or even longer to bake in the oven. Cooking them in the microwave takes only a few minutes and doesn't compromise their flavor.

1 SWEET POTATO

2 TABLESPOONS OLIVE OIL

½ ONION, CHOPPED

1 CARROT, PEELED AND CHOPPED

2 GARLIC CLOVES, MINCED

½ TEASPOON DRIED THYME

1 CUP CHOPPED KALE

SEA SALT

FRESHLY GROUND BLACK PEPPER

1. Prick the sweet potato with a fork and microwave on high until soft, about 5 minutes. Remove from the microwave and cut into ¼-inch cubes.

2. In a large nonstick sauté pan, heat the olive oil over medium-high heat. Add the onion and carrot and cook until softened, about 5 minutes. Add the garlic and thyme and cook until the garlic is fragrant, about 30 seconds.

3. Add the sweet potatoes and cook until the potatoes begin to brown, about 7 minutes. Add the kale and cook just until it wilts, 1 to 2 minutes. Season with salt and pepper. Serve immediately.

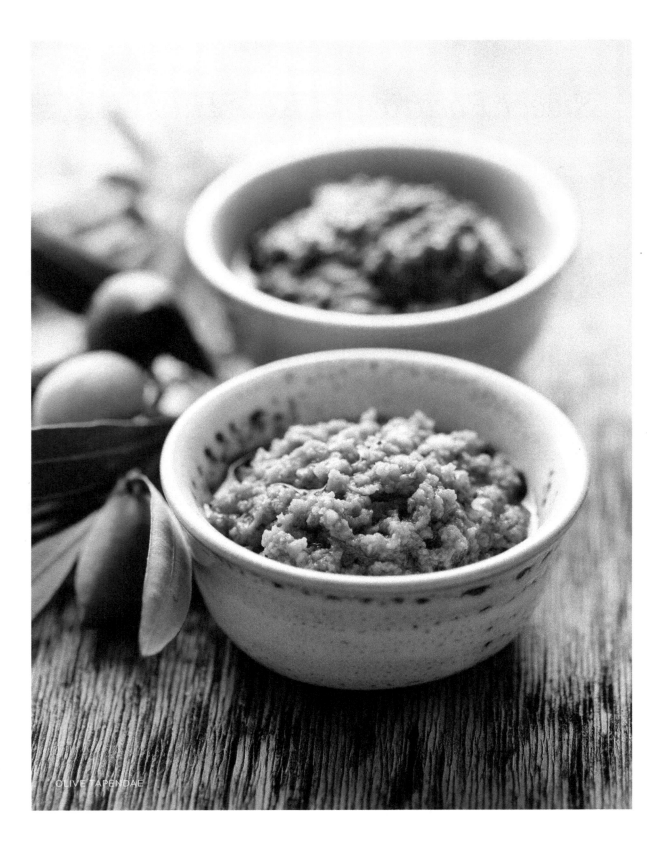

OLIVE TAPENDAE

4

Snacks

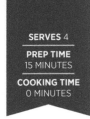

SERVES 4

PREP TIME
15 MINUTES

COOKING TIME
0 MINUTES

Jicama and Guacamole

Crunchy jicama sticks are a healthy and satisfying alternative to tortilla chips for dipping into creamy guacamole. Choose avocados that yield slightly when pressed with a thumb but aren't mushy. For the best-tasting guacamole, the flesh should be bright green without any brown spots.

Tip To store guacamole, smooth out the top so the surface is flat and pour cold water over it to completely cover. This creates a barrier that prevents oxidation and keeps your guacamole from turning an unappetizing brown color. When ready to eat, simply pour off the water, give it a stir, and you're good to go.

JUICE OF 1 LIME, OR 1 TABLESPOON
    PREPARED LIME JUICE
2 HASS AVOCADOS, PEELED, PITS
    REMOVED, AND CUT INTO CUBES
½ TEASPOON SEA SALT
½ RED ONION, MINCED

1 GARLIC CLOVE, MINCED
¼ CUP CHOPPED CILANTRO
    (OPTIONAL)
1 JICAMA BULB, PEELED AND CUT
    INTO MATCHSTICKS

1. In a medium bowl, squeeze the lime juice over the top of the avocado and sprinkle with salt. Lightly mash the avocado with a fork.

2. Stir in the onion, garlic, and cilantro, if using. Serve with slices of jicama to dip in guacamole.

3. To store, place plastic wrap over the bowl of guacamole and refrigerate. The guacamole will keep for about 2 days.

Peppers and Hummus

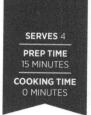

SERVES 4

PREP TIME
15 MINUTES

COOKING TIME
0 MINUTES

Homemade hummus is quick to make using canned chickpeas, and for the perfect dippers, simply slice bell peppers in a rainbow of colors. Add a handful of cured olives, some toasted pita wedges, and a bowl of Baba Ganoush (page 42) for a traditional Middle Eastern appetizer platter.

Tip For an interesting variation, substitute white beans, such as cannellini, for the chickpeas, and fresh mint, basil, or rosemary for the cumin. Garnish the white bean hummus with a splash of olive oil and some julienned sun-dried tomatoes and/or a handful of toasted pine nuts.

ONE 15-OUNCE CAN CHICKPEAS,
    DRAINED AND RINSED
JUICE OF 1 LEMON, OR 1 TABLESPOON
    PREPARED LEMON JUICE
¼ CUP TAHINI
3 TABLESPOONS OLIVE OIL

½ TEASPOON GROUND CUMIN
1 TABLESPOON WATER
¼ TEASPOON PAPRIKA
1 RED BELL PEPPER, SLICED
1 GREEN BELL PEPPER, SLICED
1 ORANGE BELL PEPPER, SLICED

1. In a food processor, combine chickpeas, lemon juice, tahini, 2 tablespoons of the olive oil, the cumin, and water. Process on high speed until blended, about 30 seconds.

2. Scoop the hummus into a bowl and drizzle with the remaining tablespoon of olive oil. Sprinkle with paprika and serve with sliced bell peppers.

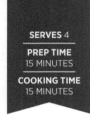
Baba Ganoush

Grilling eggplant gives it a creamy consistency and a pleasing dose of smoky flavor. Here it is puréed with tahini, lemon juice, and fresh garlic, making it a heavenly dip for pita chips or toasted pita wedges.

Tip To remove the bitterness that sometimes plagues eggplant dishes, place the peeled and sliced eggplant in a colander, sprinkle generously with salt, and let sit for about 10 minutes. Rinse away the excess salt and dry thoroughly before cooking.

2 EGGPLANTS, PEELS REMOVED AND
    SLICED
JUICE OF 1 LEMON, OR 1 TABLESPOON
    PREPARED LEMON JUICE
⅔ CUP TAHINI

2 GARLIC CLOVES, MINCED
¼ CUP MINCED FRESH PARSLEY
SEA SALT
FRESHLY GROUND BLACK PEPPER
1 BAG PITA CHIPS

1. Heat a grill on high. Place the sliced eggplant directly on the grill. Cook, turning every 5 minutes or so, until the eggplant pieces are soft, 10 to 15 minutes. Allow to cool slightly.

2. When the eggplant is cool enough to handle, cut into a fine mince finely chop the flesh.

3. In a medium bowl, combine the eggplant, lemon juice, tahini, garlic, and parsley. Whisk until well combined. Season with salt and pepper and serve with pita chips.

Olive Tapenade

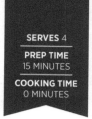
SERVES 4
PREP TIME
15 MINUTES
COOKING TIME
0 MINUTES

A rich concoction made of olives and garlic that is popular in the Mediterranean cuisines of southern France, Italy, and Greece, olive tapenade is delicious on crackers, toasted pita wedges, or baguette slices. It also makes a tasty sandwich spread. You can use green or black olives, or a combination.

½ POUND OLIVES OF YOUR CHOICE, PITTED, RINSED, AND DRAINED

2 GARLIC CLOVES, MINCED

JUICE OF ½ LEMON, OR 2 TEASPOONS PREPARED LEMON JUICE

2 TABLESPOONS OLIVE OIL

SEA SALT

FRESHLY GROUND BLACK PEPPER

CRACKERS OR SLICED BAGUETTE, FOR SERVING

1. In the bowl of a food processor, combine all the ingredients except crackers and blend for ten 1-second pulses, until everything is chopped and combined.

2. Serve the spread on crackers or baguette slices.

Salsa Fresca

With just a few ingredients, this fresh salsa is great for dipping tortilla chips and adds bright flavor to tacos and other dishes. Heirloom tomatoes are slightly sweet, lending this salsa the perfect balance of sweetness, spice, and acidity.

3 LARGE HEIRLOOM TOMATOES
    OR OTHER FRESH TOMATOES,
    CHOPPED

½ RED ONION, FINELY CHOPPED

½ BUNCH CILANTRO, CHOPPED

2 GARLIC CLOVES, MINCED

1 JALAPEÑO, MINCED

JUICE OF 1 LIME, OR 1 TABLESPOON
    PREPARED LIME JUICE

¼ CUP OLIVE OIL

SEA SALT

TORTILLA CHIPS, FOR SERVING

1. In a small bowl, combine the tomatoes, onion, cilantro, garlic, jalapeño, lime juice, and olive oil and mix well. Allow to sit at room temperature for 15 minutes. Season with salt.

2. Serve with tortilla chips. The salsa can be stored in an airtight container in the refrigerator for up to 1 week.

Spiced Nuts

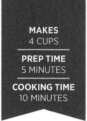
MAKES
4 CUPS

PREP TIME
5 MINUTES

COOKING TIME
10 MINUTES

Toasting nuts gives them a rich caramel flavor. The Chinese five-spice powder adds sweetness and a little bit of heat, making these an addictive snack. Keep them on hand for any time you need a quick nibble or for sprinkling on salads for extra flavor and crunch.

Tip Nuts, whether cooked or raw, can turn rancid quickly. To avoid this, store them in the freezer, where they'll stay fresh for up to 6 months.

½ POUND PECANS

½ POUND WALNUTS

1 TEASPOON SEA SALT

1 TABLESPOON DARK BROWN SUGAR

1 TEASPOON CHINESE FIVE-SPICE
    POWDER

1 TEASPOON GROUND CINNAMON

2 TABLESPOONS COCONUT OIL, MELTED

1. Preheat the oven to 350°F. Spread the pecans and walnuts in a single layer on a baking sheet. Toast until they are golden and fragrant, about 10 minutes. Watch carefully to ensure the nuts don't burn.

2. Remove from the oven and place in a medium bowl. In a separate small bowl, combine the salt, brown sugar, five-spice powder, and cinnamon.

3. Drizzle the coconut oil over the nuts and toss with the spice mix. Serve warm or store in a sealed container for up to 2 weeks.

Wasabi-Toasted Pumpkin Seeds

You can find wasabi powder in the supermarket spice aisle or in Asian grocery stores. Look for a version made with real wasabi (instead of horseradish) for the best flavor.

2 CUPS PUMPKIN SEEDS, UNSALTED
    AND DRIED

2 TEASPOONS OLIVE OIL

1 TEASPOON WASABI POWDER

2 TEASPOONS SEA SALT

1. Preheat the oven to 375°F. Toss the pumpkin seeds with olive oil and place in a single layer on a baking sheet. Bake until the seeds are crisp, 7 to 10 minutes.

2. Toss the seeds with wasabi powder and salt. Serve warm or store in an airtight container for up to 2 weeks.

Tomato and Basil Bruschetta

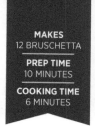

MAKES
12 BRUSCHETTA

PREP TIME
10 MINUTES

COOKING TIME
6 MINUTES

Tomatoes, basil, and olive oil are the perfect flavor combination. This recipe is at its best using in-season, organic, local—ideally homegrown or from the farmers' market—tomatoes and basil. It's like summer on toast.

Tip Make an Asian-flavored version by substituting cilantro for the basil and sesame oil for the olive oil. Top with a sprinkling of toasted sesame seeds.

3 TOMATOES, CHOPPED
¼ CUP CHOPPED FRESH BASIL
1 TABLESPOON OLIVE OIL

PINCH OF SEA SALT
1 BAGUETTE, CUT INTO 12 SLICES
1 GARLIC CLOVE, SLICED IN HALF

1. In a small bowl, combine the tomatoes, basil, olive oil, and salt and stir to mix. Set aside.

2. Preheat the oven to 425°F. Place the baguette slices in a single layer on a baking sheet and toast in the oven until brown, about 6 minutes. Flip the bread slices over once during cooking.

3. Remove from the oven and rub the bread on both sides with the sliced clove of garlic. Top with the tomato-basil mixture and serve immediately.

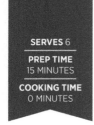
Stuffed Cherry Tomatoes

Packed with a mixture of creamy avocado, tangy lemon juice, and crunchy red peppers flavored with savory tarragon, these little bites are a delicious and impressive-looking starter.

Tip For best results, choose cherry tomatoes that are large enough to accommodate a good mouthful of the creamy filling, but small enough that they can still be eaten in one bite.

2 PINTS CHERRY TOMATOES, TOPS REMOVED AND CENTERS SCOOPED OUT

2 AVOCADOS, MASHED

JUICE OF 1 LEMON

½ RED BELL PEPPER, MINCED

4 GREEN ONIONS (WHITE AND GREEN PARTS), FINELY MINCED

1 TABLESPOON MINCED FRESH TARRAGON

PINCH OF SEA SALT

1. Place the cherry tomatoes open-side up on a platter. In a small bowl, combine the avocado, lemon juice, bell pepper, scallions, tarragon, and salt. Stir until well combined.

2. Scoop into the cherry tomatoes and serve immediately.

Asian Lettuce Rolls

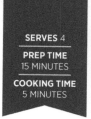

SERVES 4

PREP TIME
15 MINUTES

COOKING TIME
5 MINUTES

Crunchy lettuce leaves filled with herb- and vegetable-studded noodles are a light yet satisfying appetizer, perfect for a summer get-together. Enjoy them with a cold beer or a glass of crisp white wine.

Tip Butter lettuce has big, tender leaves that are perfect for rolls and wraps. Be sure to dry the lettuce thoroughly after washing so the rolls won't be watered down.

2 OUNCES RICE NOODLES

2 TABLESPOONS CHOPPED THAI BASIL

2 TABLESPOONS CHOPPED CILANTRO

1 GARLIC CLOVE, MINCED

1 TABLESPOON MINCED FRESH GINGER

JUICE OF ½ LIME, OR 2 TEASPOONS
    PREPARED LIME JUICE

2 TABLESPOONS SOY SAUCE

1 CUCUMBER, JULIENNED

2 CARROTS, PEELED AND JULIENNED

8 LEAVES BUTTER LETTUCE

1. Cook the rice noodles according to package directions.

2. In a small bowl, whisk together the basil, cilantro, garlic, ginger, lime juice, and soy sauce. Toss with the cooked noodles, cucumber, and carrots.

3. Divide the mixture evenly among lettuce leaves and roll. Secure with a toothpick and serve immediately.

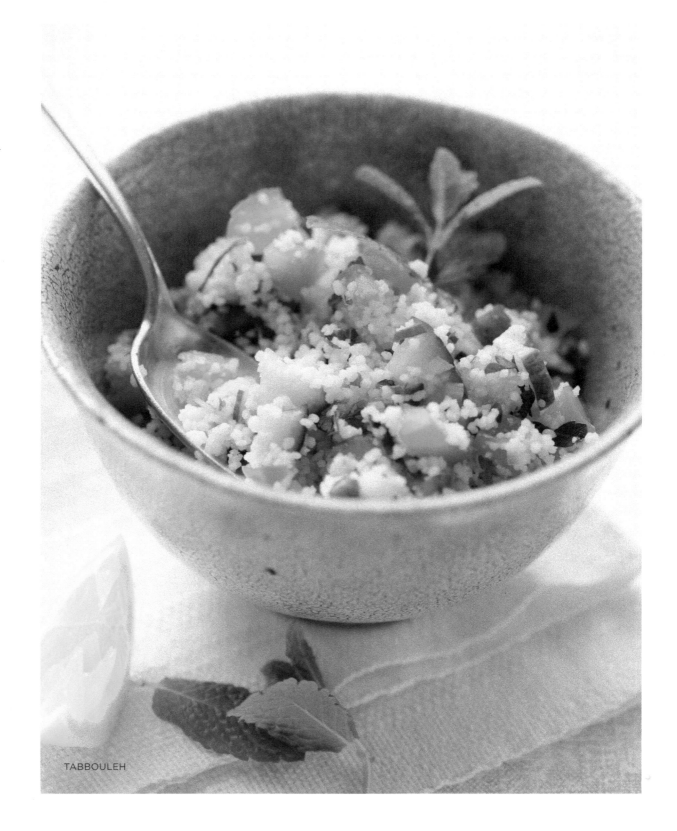

TABBOULEH

5

Salads

Ruby Grapefruit and Radicchio Salad

Ruby grapefruit adds a burst of citrus flavor to this refreshing salad. Its acidity plays nicely against the bitterness of the radicchio. Radishes add a nice crunch, and a simple lemon vinaigrette pulls it all together.

FOR THE SALAD

1 LARGE RUBY GRAPEFRUIT

1 SMALL HEAD RADICCHIO, TORN INTO
   BITE-SIZE PIECES

2 CUPS GREEN LEAF LETTUCE, TORN
   INTO BITE-SIZE PIECES

2 CUPS BABY SPINACH

1 BUNCH WATERCRESS

4 TO 6 RADISHES, SLICED PAPER-THIN

FOR THE DRESSING

JUICE OF 1 LEMON

2 TEASPOONS AGAVE

1 TEASPOON WHITE WINE VINEGAR

½ TEASPOON SEA SALT

½ TEASPOON FRESHLY GROUND
   BLACK PEPPER

¼ CUP EXTRA-VIRGIN OLIVE OIL

1. **To make the salad:** Cut both ends off of the grapefruit, stand it on a cutting board on one of the flat sides, and, using a sharp knife, cut away the peel and all of the white pith. Remove the individual segments by slicing between the membrane and fruit on each side of each segment, dropping the fruit into a large salad bowl as you go.

2. Add the radicchio, lettuce, spinach, watercress, and radishes to the bowl and toss well.

3. **To make the dressing:** Whisk together the lemon juice, agave, vinegar, salt, and pepper. Slowly whisk in the olive oil until the mixture is well combined and emulsified.

4. Toss the salad with the dressing and serve immediately.

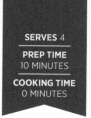

Apple and Ginger Slaw

This fresh, crispy slaw is bright with the flavors of apples and ginger. Use sweet-tart apples such as Granny Smith or Honeycrisp for just the right crunch and balance of flavors. Serve it alongside roasted vegetables or on top of spicy Asian-flavored veggie burgers.

Tip Red cabbage is particularly stunning in this salad, but if it's unavailable, you can substitute regular green cabbage and add a handful of julienned bright pink radishes or thinly sliced red onions for a dash of color.

2 TABLESPOONS OLIVE OIL

JUICE OF 1 LEMON, OR 2 TABLE-
  SPOONS PREPARED LEMON JUICE

1 TEASPOON GRATED FRESH GINGER

PINCH OF SEA SALT

2 APPLES, PEELED AND JULIENNED

4 CUPS SHREDDED RED CABBAGE

1. In a small bowl, whisk together the olive oil, lemon juice, ginger, and salt and set aside.

2. In a large bowl, combine the apples and cabbage. Toss with the vinaigrette and serve immediately. Store leftovers in an airtight container in the refrigerator for up to 3 days.

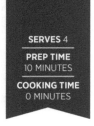
Spinach and Pomegranate Salad

This colorful salad is loaded with antioxidants. The sweet-tangy balsamic vinaigrette is a perfect bridge for the sweet berries, tart pomegranate seeds, and herby spinach. Red onions add a welcome bite, and pecans a nice crunch.

Tip You could substitute just about any leafy salad green for the spinach in this recipe. Try peppery arugula or delicate Little Gem lettuce for a change of pace.

10 OUNCES BABY SPINACH

SEEDS FROM 1 POMEGRANATE

1 CUP FRESH BLACKBERRIES

¼ RED ONION, THINLY SLICED

½ CUP CHOPPED PECANS

¼ CUP BALSAMIC VINEGAR

¾ CUP OLIVE OIL

½ TEASPOON SEA SALT

½ TEASPOON FRESHLY GROUND
BLACK PEPPER

1. In a large bowl, combine the spinach, pomegranate seeds, blackberries, red onion, and pecans.

2. In a small bowl, whisk together the vinegar, olive oil, salt, and pepper. Toss with the salad and serve immediately.

Pear and Arugula Salad

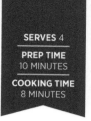

SERVES 4

PREP TIME
10 MINUTES

COOKING TIME
8 MINUTES

Sweet and tender pears, peppery arugula, and crunchy pecans make for a lovely fall salad. For best results, use fresh pears that are ripe but still have a bit of crunch. Bosc or Bartlett pears are good choices.

Tip Radicchio, a dark purple leafy vegetable with a pleasingly bitter bite, can be substituted for the arugula. Other nice variations include chopped hazelnuts or walnuts instead of pecans, and hazelnut oil or walnut oil in place of olive oil.

¼ CUP CHOPPED PECANS

10 OUNCES ARUGULA

2 PEARS, THINLY SLICED

1 TABLESPOON FINELY MINCED
   SHALLOT

2 TABLESPOONS CHAMPAGNE
   VINEGAR

2 TABLESPOONS OLIVE OIL

¼ TEASPOON SEA SALT

¼ TEASPOON FRESHLY GROUND
   BLACK PEPPER

¼ TEASPOON DIJON MUSTARD

1. Preheat the oven to 350°F. Spread the pecans in a single layer on a baking sheet. Toast in the preheated oven until fragrant, about 6 minutes. Remove from the oven and let cool.

2. In a large bowl, toss the pecans, arugula, and pears.

3. In a small bowl, whisk together the shallot, vinegar, olive oil, salt, pepper, and mustard. Toss with the salad and serve immediately.

Apple and Fennel Salad

Though they may seem like odd bedfellows, apples and fennel are both at their seasonal peak in the fall and pair surprisingly well together. Choose a crisp, tart green apple such as Granny Smith, which provides a bright counterpoint to the anise flavor of the fennel.

Tip When you buy fennel bulbs, try to choose ones with their leafy tops still attached. They're sure to be fresh and you can mince the licorice-scented leaves to use in a salad dressing or as a flavorful garnish.

5 APPLES, THINLY SLICED

JUICE OF ½ LEMON

2 FENNEL BULBS, THINLY SLICED

2 STALKS CELERY, THINLY SLICED

½ BUNCH FRESH PARSLEY, CHOPPED

2 TABLESPOONS MINCED FENNEL
 FRONDS

2 TABLESPOONS APPLE CIDER
 VINEGAR

¼ CUP OLIVE OIL

¼ TEASPOON SEA SALT

¼ TEASPOON FRESHLY GROUND
 BLACK PEPPER

1. In a large bowl, toss the apples with the lemon juice. Add the sliced fennel, celery, and parsley and toss to combine.

2. In a small bowl, whisk together the fennel fronds, vinegar, olive oil, salt, and pepper. Toss with the salad and serve immediately.

German Potato Salad

SERVES 8

PREP TIME
15 MINUTES

COOKING TIME
15 MINUTES

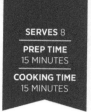

This classic potato salad is dressed with vinaigrette, making it both lighter and brighter than its mayonnaise-heavy counterparts. Crunchy red onions and vibrant green chives add both visual and textural interest as well as flavor. For the best result, use a good-quality extra-virgin olive oil.

Tip This potato salad gets better with time as the starchy potatoes soak up the flavorful dressing. Make it a day or two ahead and refrigerate in an airtight container. Bring it to room temperature before serving.

8 RED POTATOES, CUT INTO
    1-INCH CHUNKS

3 TEASPOONS SEA SALT

1 RED ONION, FINELY CHOPPED

¼ CUP OLIVE OIL

2 TABLESPOONS DIJON MUSTARD

2 TABLESPOONS RED WINE VINEGAR

½ TEASPOON FRESHLY GROUND
    BLACK PEPPER

3 TABLESPOONS MINCED CHIVES

1. In a large pot filled with water, combine the potatoes and 2 teaspoons of the salt. Boil until the potatoes are tender, about 10 minutes. Place in a bowl with the red onion.

2. In a small saucepan over medium heat, whisk together the olive oil, mustard, vinegar, the remaining 1 teaspoon salt, and the pepper.

3. Heat until warm, then remove from heat. Toss with the potatoes and onion. Stir in the chives and serve warm.

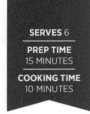

SERVES 6

PREP TIME
15 MINUTES

COOKING TIME
10 MINUTES

Tabbouleh

This flavorful Middle Eastern salad contains a beautiful mix of fragrant herbs, including mint, basil, and parsley. Using fresh herbs is an absolute must here. For a twist, this version substitutes quick-cooking couscous for the traditional bulgur.

Tip To make this into a gluten-free recipe, substitute quinoa for the couscous. Just follow the cooking instructions on the quinoa package to prepare it.

1⅓ CUPS COUSCOUS

2 CUPS VEGETABLE STOCK

1 TOMATO, CHOPPED

1 CUCUMBER, CHOPPED

¼ CUP OLIVE OIL

2 TABLESPOONS LEMON JUICE

2 TABLESPOONS CHOPPED
    FRESH BASIL

2 TABLESPOONS CHOPPED FRESH
    PARSLEY

1 TABLESPOON CHOPPED FRESH MINT

½ TEASPOON SEA SALT

¼ TEASPOON FRESHLY GROUND
    BLACK PEPPER

1. In a large saucepan over medium high heat, bring the vegetable stock to a boil. Add the couscous and remove from the heat. Cover the pan and allow it to sit until the couscous is fluffy, about 5 minutes. Let cool completely.

2. In a medium bowl, combine the cooled couscous with the tomato and cucumber.

3. In a small bowl, whisk together the olive oil, lemon juice, basil, parsley, mint, salt, and pepper. Toss with the couscous and vegetables. Serve immediately.

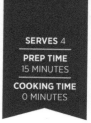
Kale and Root Vegetable Salad

This is the best kind of just-back-from-the-farmers'-market salad. Kale and root vegetables, like carrots and turnips, are all at their peak during the fall harvest season, when you'll find piles of them at your local market. The result is a rainbow of a salad that is simply packed with nutrition and flavor.

1½ POUNDS KALE, CUT INTO
    THIN STRIPS
2 CARROTS, PEELED AND GRATED
1 TURNIP, PEELED AND GRATED
4 RADISHES, GRATED
3 GREEN ONIONS (WHITE AND GREEN
    PARTS), CUT INTO THIN STRIPS
2 TABLESPOONS OLIVE OIL

1 TABLESPOON LEMON JUICE
ZEST OF ½ LEMON
2 TEASPOONS AGAVE
½ TEASPOON SEA SALT
¼ TEASPOON FRESHLY GROUND
    BLACK PEPPER
PINCH OF CAYENNE PEPPER
    (OPTIONAL)

1. In a large bowl, combine the kale, carrots, turnip, radishes, and green onions.

2. In a small bowl, whisk together the olive oil, lemon juice, lemon zest, agave, salt, pepper, and cayenne, if using. Toss with the kale mixture and serve immediately.

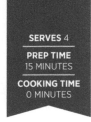

Brown Rice and Pepper Salad

Crunchy, colorful carrots and peppers tossed with Asian flavorings make this an interesting twist on the classic rice salad. Serve it at a picnic, a barbecue, or any time you want a cold but filling side dish.

Tip This salad is quick to make when you use leftover rice. You can cook a large batch of rice and refrigerate or freeze it in preportioned quantities, or you can purchase pre-cooked, frozen rice at the supermarket. If using frozen rice, thaw it thoroughly before proceeding with the recipe.

2 CUPS PREPARED BROWN RICE

½ RED ONION, DICED

1 RED BELL PEPPER, DICED

1 ORANGE BELL PEPPER, DICED

1 CARROT, DICED

¼ CUP OLIVE OIL

2 TABLESPOONS UNSEASONED
     RICE VINEGAR

1 TABLESPOON SOY SAUCE

1 GARLIC CLOVE, MINCED

1 TABLESPOON GRATED FRESH GINGER

¼ TEASPOON SEA SALT

¼ TEASPOON FRESHLY GROUND
     BLACK PEPPER

1. In a large bowl, combine the rice, onion, bell peppers, and carrot.

2. In a small bowl, whisk together the olive oil, rice vinegar, soy sauce, garlic, ginger, salt, and pepper. Toss with the rice mixture and serve immediately.

Three-Bean Salad

SERVES 4

PREP TIME
10 MINUTES

COOKING TIME
0 MINUTES

This salad—a favorite standby at backyard barbecues and summer picnics—is easy to assemble and is best made well in advance, as it gets better with time. Allow it to sit for several hours, or even as long as a few days, before serving so that the flavors can fully develop.

ONE 15-OUNCE CAN CHICKPEAS,
    DRAINED AND RINSED
ONE 15-OUNCE CAN KIDNEY BEANS,
    DRAINED AND RINSED
ONE 15-OUNCE CAN CANNELLINI
    BEANS, DRAINED AND RINSED
1 RED ONION, FINELY CHOPPED
1 CUP FINELY CHOPPED FRESH
    PARSLEY
⅓ CUP WHITE WINE VINEGAR

2 TABLESPOONS AGAVE
¼ CUP OLIVE OIL
1 TEASPOON CHOPPED FRESH
    ROSEMARY
1 TEASPOON SEA SALT
¼ TEASPOON FRESHLY GROUND
    BLACK PEPPER
PINCH OF CAYENNE PEPPER
    (OPTIONAL)

1. In a large bowl, combine the beans, onion, and parsley and toss to mix.

2. In a small bowl, whisk together the vinegar, agave, olive oil, rosemary, salt, pepper, and cayenne, if using. Toss with the bean mixture. Refrigerate for several hours before serving to allow the flavors to blend.

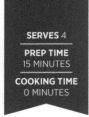
SERVES 4

PREP TIME
15 MINUTES

COOKING TIME
0 MINUTES

Satsuma, Grapefruit, and Pomegranate Salad

Satsuma oranges are sweet and easy to peel, and their small wedges are perfectly bite-size. Along with grapefruit and pomegranate, they make a bright, colorful salad that works equally well as a side dish, breakfast, or dessert.

Tip If you can't find satsumas, substitute clementines, mandarins, or tangerines. Even small, juicy oranges will work, but you'll want to remove the seeds from the wedges before adding them to the salad.

10 SATSUMA ORANGES, PEELED
AND SECTIONED

SEEDS OF 1 POMEGRANATE

1 PINK GRAPEFRUIT, PEELED AND
THINLY SLICED

JUICE OF 1 ORANGE

In a large bowl, combine the oranges, pomegranate seeds, and grapefruit. Pour the orange juice over the top and toss to combine. Refrigerate for 2 hours to allow the flavors to blend before serving.

NOTES

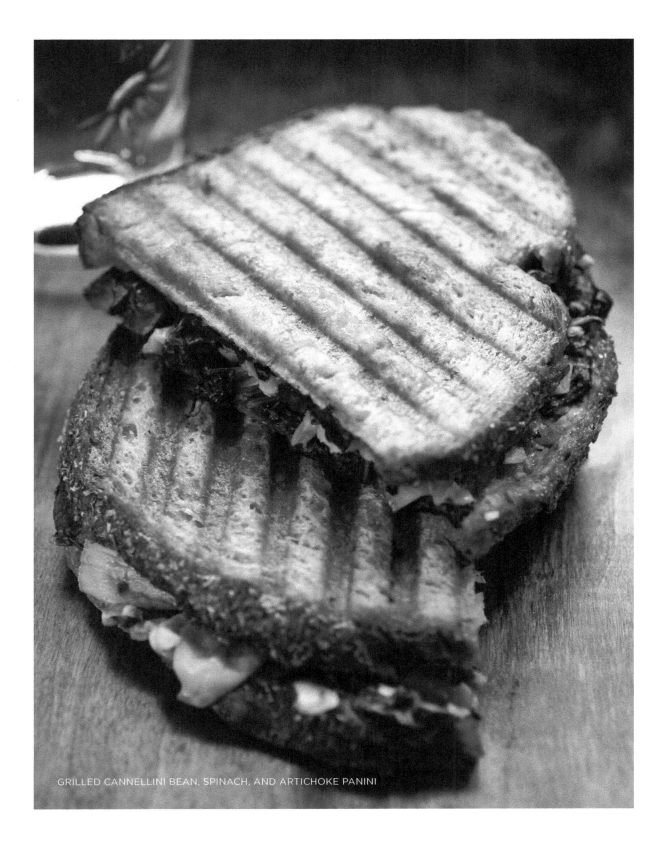

GRILLED CANNELLINI BEAN, SPINACH, AND ARTICHOKE PANINI

6

Sandwiches

Avocado and Spicy Sprout Sandwich

Spicy sprouts add zip to this sandwich and are a perfect counterpoint to the creamy avocado. Zesty Dijon mustard, tangy lemon, and a kick of cayenne make this sandwich special. Use hearty multigrain or seeded bread for a satisfying lunch.

4 SLICES BREAD

2 TABLESPOONS DIJON MUSTARD

1 AVOCADO, PEELED AND PITTED

JUICE AND ZEST OF ½ LEMON

PINCH OF CAYENNE PEPPER

½ TEASPOON SEA SALT

¼ TEASPOON FRESHLY GROUND
   BLACK PEPPER

2 CUPS SPICY SPROUTS, SUCH AS
   RADISH OR ARUGULA SPROUTS

4 SLICES TOMATO

1. Spread each of two slices of bread with 1 tablespoon Dijon mustard.

2. In a small bowl, combine the avocado, lemon juice, lemon zest, cayenne, salt, and black pepper and mash with a fork.

3. Spread the avocado mixture evenly on the two remaining slices of bread. Top each with 1 cup of spicy sprouts and two slices of tomato. Top with Dijon-spread bread. Serve immediately.

Grilled Portobello and Red Pepper Sandwich

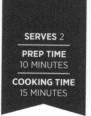

SERVES 2

PREP TIME
10 MINUTES

COOKING TIME
15 MINUTES

Portobello mushrooms become easily waterlogged. Instead of rinsing them, clean them with a mushroom brush or paper towel. Then use the edge of a spoon to scrape out the black gills before slicing.

4 SLICES BREAD

2 TABLESPOONS DIJON MUSTARD

2 TABLESPOONS OLIVE OIL

2 PORTOBELLO MUSHROOMS, CUT
    INTO ¼-INCH SLICES

1 RED BELL PEPPER, CUT INTO 4 SLICES

SEA SALT

FRESHLY GROUND BLACK PEPPER

½ CUP ARUGULA

1. Spread two slices of bread with Dijon mustard.

2. Set a grill to high or place a grill pan on high heat. Brush olive oil onto the mushrooms and bell peppers and grill, turning occasionally, until soft. The mushrooms will take approximately 5 minutes, while the bell peppers will take about 10 minutes.

3. Remove the vegetables from the heat and sprinkle them with salt and pepper. Place on the two remaining slices of bread. Top each with ¼ cup arugula and then top with Dijon-spread bread. Serve immediately.

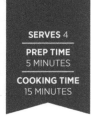

Italian Eggplant Sandwich

A simple pesto made with red bell peppers, spinach, pine nuts, and olive oil gives this sandwich unmistakable Italian flavor. For just the right combination of textures—creamy eggplant and crunchy bread—be sure to toast the ciabatta rolls before assembling the sandwiches.

Tip Salting eggplant to draw out the moisture before cooking ensures a nice texture and also eliminates the bitterness eggplant sometimes has. Place the sliced eggplant in a colander, sprinkle generously with salt, and let sit for about 10 minutes. Rinse away the excess salt and dry thoroughly before cooking.

4 CIABATTA ROLLS, HALVED
    LENGTHWISE
1 EGGPLANT, CUT INTO 4 SLICES
¼ CUP PLUS 2 TABLESPOONS
    OLIVE OIL
½ CUP FRESH BASIL
½ CUP BABY SPINACH

½ CUP PINE NUTS
¼ CUP JARRED ROASTED RED
    BELL PEPPERS, DRAINED
4 GARLIC CLOVES
SEA SALT
FRESHLY GROUND BLACK PEPPER

1. Preheat the oven to 350°F, and preheat a grill to high or set a grill pan over high heat. Place split the ciabatta rolls cut-side up on a baking sheet and toast in the preheated oven for about 8 minutes, until well-toasted and crisp.

2. Meanwhile, brush the eggplant with 2 tablespoons of the olive oil and grill until soft, 4 to 5 minutes per side.

3. In a food processor, combine the basil, spinach, pine nuts, roasted bell peppers, garlic, and the remaining ¼ cup olive oil until the basil and spinach are finely chopped and the mixture is well combined. Season with salt and pepper. Spread pesto on the toasted rolls and top with the roasted eggplant. Serve immediately.

Veggie Muffaletta

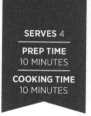
You can buy tapenade premade or make it yourself using the Olive Tapenade recipe from this book (page 43). Make the sandwich a few hours in advance, wrap it tightly, and let it rest in the refrigerator at least 15 minutes to allow the flavors to blend.

1 ROUND SOURDOUGH LOAF

2 TABLESPOONS OLIVE OIL

1 GREEN BELL PEPPER, SLICED

1 RED BELL PEPPER, SLICED

1 YELLOW BELL PEPPER, SLICED

1 SWEET ONION, SLICED

2 GARLIC CLOVES, MINCED

½ TEASPOON SEA SALT

1 CUP PREMADE OLIVE TAPENADE

1. Cut the sourdough loaf in half lengthwise and scoop out about half the bread from the center of each side.

2. In a large sauté pan, heat the olive oil over medium-high heat until it shimmers. Add the bell peppers and onion and cook until soft, about 10 minutes. Add the garlic and cook until it is fragrant, about 30 seconds. Add the salt and stir to combine. Remove from the heat.

3. Spread the tapenade in half of the scooped-out bread. Top with the vegetables and the other half of the sourdough loaf.

4. Wrap tightly in plastic and refrigerate for up to 2 to 3 hours before serving so the bread can soak up the juices from the vegetables and tapenade. Unwrap and slice into four wedges to serve.

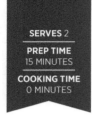

SERVES 2

PREP TIME
15 MINUTES

COOKING TIME
0 MINUTES

Black Bean and Avocado Wraps

Protein-packed black beans, creamy avocado, and spicy salsa make this wrap a filling and satisfying lunch. Mashing the avocado with the lime juice keeps it bright green. Use a premade salsa or make your own using the recipe for Salsa Fresca in this book (page 44).

ONE 15-OUNCE CAN BLACK BEANS, DRAINED AND RINSED
¼ CUP PREMADE SALSA
½ TEASPOON SEA SALT
1 AVOCADO, PITTED AND SLICED
1 GARLIC CLOVE, MINCED

JUICE OF 1 LIME
4 WHOLE-WHEAT VEGAN TORTILLAS
1 TOMATO, CHOPPED
1 CUP CHOPPED ROMAINE LETTUCE
PICKLED JALAPEÑOS (OPTIONAL)

1. In a small bowl, mash the beans with a fork. Add the salsa and salt and stir to combine.

2. In another small bowl, mash the avocado with the garlic and lime juice.

3. Spread the bean-salsa mixture on tortillas and top with the avocado mixture. Add the tomato, lettuce, and jalapeño, if using. Roll each into a wrap and serve immediately.

Mediterranean Pita with Red Onion Quick Pickle

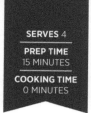

SERVES 4

PREP TIME
15 MINUTES

COOKING TIME
0 MINUTES

The quick pickle of red onions gives this sandwich a bright acidity and a lovely crunch. Quickly pickling onions can make for a great addition to other sandwiches and salads as well. You can use purchased hummus or make it yourself using the Peppers and Hummus recipe from this book (page 41).

½ RED ONION, THINLY SLICED

¼ CUP RED WINE VINEGAR

2 TABLESPOONS SEA SALT

2 TABLESPOONS SUGAR

2 WHOLE-WHEAT PITAS, HALVED

1 CUP HUMMUS

1 CUCUMBER, CHOPPED

1 TOMATO, CHOPPED

1 RED BELL PEPPER, CHOPPED

1. Place the onion in a small bowl. In a separate small bowl, whisk together the vinegar, salt, and sugar. Pour the vinegar mixture over the onion and allow to rest at room temperature for 30 minutes. Drain before using.

2. Open the pitas and spread ¼ cup hummus in each. Add the cucumber, tomato, bell pepper, and pickled onion. Serve immediately.

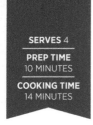
Grilled Cannellini Bean, Spinach, and Artichoke Panini

These grilled sandwiches are loaded with flavor from the garlic, fresh thyme, lemon juice, and artichoke hearts. The white beans add plenty of protein and a creaminess that really pulls the sandwich together.

Tip If you don't have a panini press, you can place a frying pan—or better yet, a cast-iron skillet—on top of the sandwiches and weigh it down with something solid, like a heavy can, while they are cooking.

ONE 15-OUNCE CAN CANNELLINI
    BEANS, DRAINED AND RINSED
2 GARLIC CLOVES, FINELY MINCED
½ TEASPOON SEA SALT
1 TABLESPOON CHOPPED
    FRESH THYME

ZEST AND JUICE OF 1 LEMON
8 SLICES BREAD
1 JAR ARTICHOKE HEARTS, DRAINED
½ CUP BABY SPINACH LEAVES
2 TABLESPOONS OLIVE OIL

1. In a medium bowl, lightly mash beans with garlic, salt, thyme, lemon juice, and lemon zest. Spread the mixture evenly over four slices of bread. Top with the artichoke hearts and spinach leaves, divided evenly among the sandwiches. Top with the remaining slices of bread. Brush the outside of the bread with olive oil.

2. Heat a large frying pan or panini press over medium-high heat. If using a panini press, cook for about 7 minutes. If using a frying pan, cook for about 7 minutes per side. Serve immediately.

Italian Hoagie

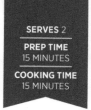

SERVES 2
PREP TIME
15 MINUTES
COOKING TIME
15 MINUTES

This delicious sandwich is literally dripping with Italian flavor. Mushrooms, bell peppers, zucchini, and onions are sautéed with garlic and olive oil, then piled onto toasted hoagie rolls. Using prepared Italian salad dressing as a sandwich spread adds taste in a snap.

Tip For best results, after adding the mushrooms to the pan, allow them to develop flavor by sitting in the pan without stirring for 3 to 4 minutes. Then continue cooking, stirring occasionally, until the mushrooms brown.

2 HOAGIE ROLLS

¼ CUP PREPARED ITALIAN SALAD DRESSING

2 TABLESPOONS OLIVE OIL

½ RED BELL PEPPER, SLICED

½ GREEN BELL PEPPER, SLICED

½ SWEET ONION, SLICED

12 CREMINI MUSHROOMS, SLICED

1 ZUCCHINI, SLICED

3 GARLIC CLOVES, SLICED

SEA SALT

FRESHLY GROUND BLACK PEPPER

½ TEASPOON RED PEPPER FLAKES (OPTIONAL)

1 TOMATO, SLICED

1. Slice the hoagie rolls lengthwise and spread with the Italian salad dressing.

2. In a large sauté pan, heat the olive oil until it shimmers. Add the bell peppers and onion and cook until soft, about 5 minutes. Add the mushrooms and zucchini and cook until all the vegetables are soft, about 7 minutes more. Add the garlic, season with salt and pepper and add the red pepper flakes, if using, and cook until the garlic is fragrant, about 30 seconds.

3. Spoon the bell pepper mixture onto hoagie rolls and top with the tomato slices. Serve immediately.

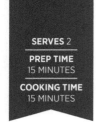

Tempeh Reuben Sandwich

Vegan deli food never tasted so good. Using store-bought tempeh, jarred sauerkraut, and prepared French dressing makes these Reuben sandwiches quick and easy to prepare—and you'll swear the flavor is right out of a New York deli.

¼ CUP SOY SAUCE

½ ONION, MINCED

2 GARLIC CLOVES, MINCED

4 OUNCES TEMPEH, SLICED

4 SLICES RYE BREAD

2 TABLESPOONS PREPARED
FRENCH DRESSING

½ CUP PREPARED SAUERKRAUT

4 DILL PICKLES, SLICED

1. In a medium saucepan over medium heat, simmer the soy sauce, onion, garlic, and tempeh slices for about 10 minutes. Remove the tempeh from the marinade and set aside.

2. Meanwhile, preheat the oven to 350°F and toast the bread, about 5 minutes on each side.

3. Spread two slices of bread with French dressing. Top with sliced tempeh, sauerkraut, pickles, and the remaining slice of bread. Serve immediately.

Seitan Barbecue Sandwich

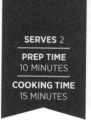

Here is the vegan answer to a classic Southern pulled-pork sandwich. Slathered in smoky barbecue sauce and piled high with a crunchy cabbage slaw, this sandwich and a cold beer are all you need on a warm summer evening.

½ CUP PREPARED BARBECUE SAUCE

2 CUPS SEITAN

1 TABLESPOON OLIVE OIL

½ TABLESPOON APPLE CIDER VINEGAR

1 CUP SHREDDED NAPA CABBAGE

1 CARROT, PEELED AND GRATED

½ ONION, MINCED

2 HAMBURGER BUNS

1. In a small saucepan over low heat, heat the barbecue sauce until it is warm. In a medium saucepan, boil the seitan in water for 5 minutes and drain. Mix the seitan with the warm barbecue sauce.

2. Meanwhile, in a medium bowl, whisk together the olive oil and vinegar. Add the cabbage, carrot, and onion and toss to combine. Top the lower half of the hamburger buns with the seitan mixture, the cabbage mixture, and the bun tops. Serve immediately.

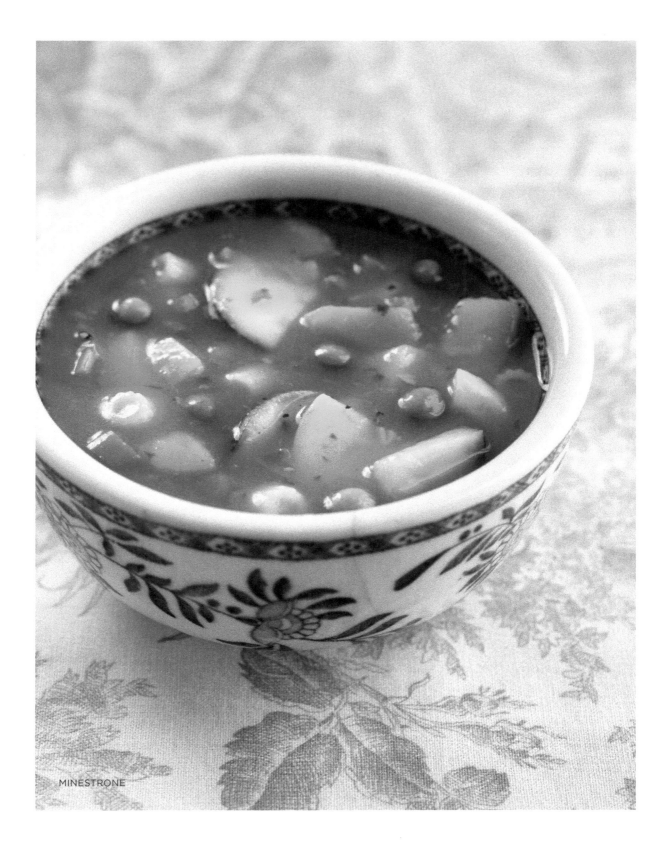

MINESTRONE

7

Soups, Stews, and Chilies

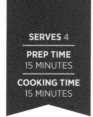
Coconut and Curry Soup

Rich coconut milk and spicy curry are studded with vegetables to make a comforting and flavorful soup. Add cooked rice or eggless noodles in the second step of the recipe to turn it into a filling one-pot meal.

1 TABLESPOON COCONUT OIL

½ ONION, THINLY SLICED

1 CARROT, PEELED AND JULIENNED

½ CUP SLICED SHIITAKE MUSHROOMS

3 GARLIC CLOVES, MINCED

ONE 14-OUNCE CAN COCONUT MILK

1 CUP VEGETABLE STOCK

JUICE FROM 1 LIME, OR 2 TEASPOONS
    LIME JUICE

½ TEASPOON SEA SALT

2 TEASPOONS CURRY POWDER

1. In a large soup pot, heat the coconut oil over medium-high heat until it shimmers. Add the onion, carrot, and mushrooms and cook until soft, about 7 minutes. Stir in the garlic and cook until it is fragrant, about 30 seconds.

2. Add the coconut milk, vegetable stock, lime juice, salt, and curry powder and heat through. Serve immediately.

Root Vegetable Soup

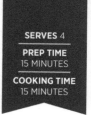

SERVES 4

PREP TIME
15 MINUTES

COOKING TIME
15 MINUTES

This recipe requires you to grate or julienne vegetables so they cook more quickly. When processing hot foods in the food processor, be sure to protect your hand with a folded towel to avoid burns, and allow steam to escape through the top hatch.

2 TABLESPOONS OLIVE OIL

1 ONION, DICED

3 GARLIC CLOVES, MINCED

1 CARROT, JULIENNED OR GRATED

1 RUTABAGA, JULIENNED OR GRATED

1 PARSNIP, JULIENNED OR GRATED

1 RED POTATO, JULIENNED OR GRATED

5 CUPS VEGETABLE STOCK

2 TEASPOONS DRIED THYME

SEA SALT

FRESHLY GROUND BLACK PEPPER

1. In a large soup pot, heat the olive oil over medium-high heat until it shimmers. Add the onion and cook until it softens, about 5 minutes. Add the garlic and cook until it is fragrant, about 30 seconds. Add the carrot, rutabaga, parsnip, potato, vegetable stock, and thyme. Cover and boil until vegetables soften, about 10 minutes.

2. Remove from the heat. Using a food processor or blender, purée the soup in batches. Season with salt and pepper. Serve immediately.

Minestrone

This classic Italian soup is full of vegetables and beans. Feel free to add or substitute whatever vegetables or beans you have on hand, as this soup is quite versatile. If you want a heartier soup, add a few cups of cooked pasta before serving.

2 TABLESPOONS OLIVE OIL

½ ONION, DICED

1 CARROT, PEELED AND DICED

1 STALK CELERY, DICED

4 GARLIC CLOVES, MINCED

5 CUPS VEGETABLE STOCK

1 ZUCCHINI, DICED

ONE 15-OUNCE CAN KIDNEY BEANS,
    DRAINED AND RINSED

ONE 15-OUNCE CAN CHOPPED
    TOMATOES WITH LIQUID, OR
    2 FRESH TOMATOES, PEELED
    AND CHOPPED

2 TEASPOONS ITALIAN SEASONING

SEA SALT

FRESHLY GROUND PEPPER

1. In a large soup pot, heat the olive oil over medium-high heat until it shimmers. Add the onion, carrot, and celery and cook until vegetables soften, about 5 minutes. Add the garlic and cook until it is fragrant, about 30 seconds.

2. Add the vegetable stock, zucchini, kidney beans, tomatoes, and Italian seasoning. Simmer the soup until the vegetables are soft, about 10 minutes. Season with salt and pepper and serve immediately.

Four-Bean Chili

SERVES 6

PREP TIME
10 MINUTES

COOKING TIME
15 MINUTES

Fortified with black, kidney, pinto, and white beans, this chili is packed with protein. Garlic and chili powder add irresistible flavor. For extra heat, you can add a pinch of cayenne pepper or some chopped chipotle chiles.

Tip Ro-Tel tomatoes and peppers (in the canned tomato section of the supermarket) add spice to this chili. If you can't find them, substitute two cans of regular diced tomatoes and a can of diced, roasted green chiles.

2 TABLESPOONS OLIVE OIL

1 ONION, CHOPPED

4 GARLIC CLOVES, MINCED

ONE 15-OUNCE CAN BLACK BEANS,
    DRAINED AND RINSED

ONE 15-OUNCE CAN KIDNEY BEANS,
    DRAINED AND RINSED

ONE 15-OUNCE CAN PINTO BEANS,
    DRAINED AND RINSED

ONE 15-OUNCE CAN WHITE BEANS,
    DRAINED AND RINSED

TWO 15-OUNCE CANS RO-TEL
    ROASTED TOMATOES
    AND PEPPERS

2 CUPS VEGETABLE STOCK

3 TABLESPOONS CHILI POWDER

1 TEASPOON SEA SALT

1. In a large pot, heat the olive oil over medium-high heat until it shimmers. Add the onion and cook until it softens, about 5 minutes. Add the garlic and cook until it is fragrant, about 30 seconds.

2. Add the beans, tomatoes and peppers, vegetable stock, chili powder, and salt. Cook, stirring occasionally, until heated through, about 10 minutes. Serve immediately.

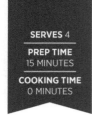
Spicy Gazpacho

A cool gazpacho makes a perfect lunch on a blazing-hot summer day. It's a good thing that tomatoes and herbs are at their peak during the hot summer months, because using fresh, very ripe, flavorful tomatoes and fresh herbs is an absolute must here.

Tip Everyone has a different tolerance for spice. Start with a small amount of cayenne pepper and then adjust until you reach the desired level of heat.

1 TABLESPOON OLIVE OIL

3 CUPS VEGETABLE JUICE,
    SUCH AS V8

1 RED ONION, DICED

3 TOMATOES, CHOPPED

1 RED BELL PEPPER, DICED

2 GARLIC CLOVES, MINCED

JUICE OF 1 LEMON

2 TABLESPOONS CHOPPED
    FRESH BASIL

¼ TO ½ TEASPOON CAYENNE PEPPER

SEA SALT

FRESHLY GROUND BLACK PEPPER

1. In a blender or a food processor, combine the olive oil, vegetable juice, all but ½ cup of the onion, all but ½ cup of the tomato, all but ½ cup of the bell pepper, the garlic, lemon juice, basil, and cayenne. Season with salt and pepper and process until smooth.

2. Stir the reserved ½ cup onion, ½ cup tomatoes, and ½ cup bell pepper into the processed ingredients and refrigerate for 1 hour. Serve chilled.

Easy Corn Chowder

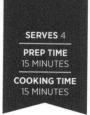

SERVES 4

PREP TIME
15 MINUTES

COOKING TIME
15 MINUTES

While fresh, in-season vegetables always offer the absolute best flavor, this chowder is fantastic whether you use fresh, frozen, or even canned corn, so you can enjoy it any time of year. If you like your chowder spicier, feel free to add more Sriracha sauce, or pass the bottle at the table and let everyone spice their own bowl.

2 TABLESPOONS OLIVE OIL OR OTHER
    VEGETABLE OIL, SUCH AS
    COCONUT OIL
1 ONION, CHOPPED
1 CUP CHOPPED FENNEL BULB
    OR CELERY
2 CARROTS, PEELED AND CHOPPED
1 RED BELL PEPPER, FINELY CHOPPED
¼ CUP ALL-PURPOSE FLOUR
6 CUPS VEGETABLE STOCK

2 CUPS FRESH OR CANNED CORN
2 CUPS CUBED RED POTATO
1 CUP UNSWEETENED ALMOND MILK
    OR OTHER UNSWEETENED NUT
    OR GRAIN MILK
½ TEASPOON SRIRACHA SAUCE OR
    CHILI PASTE (OPTIONAL)
SEA SALT
FRESHLY GROUND BLACK PEPPER

1. In a large pot, heat the olive oil over medium-high heat until it shimmers. Add the onion, fennel, carrots, and bell pepper and cook, stirring occasionally, until the vegetables soften, about 3 minutes.

2. Sprinkle the flour over the vegetables and continue to cook, stirring constantly, for about 2 minutes.

3. Stir in the vegetable stock, using a spoon to scrape any bits of flour or vegetables from the bottom of the pan. Continue stirring until the liquid comes to a boil and the soup begins to thicken.

4. Lower the heat to medium. Add the corn, potatoes, almond milk, and Sriracha, if using. Simmer until the potatoes are soft, about 10 minutes. Season with salt and pepper. Serve hot.

Potato and Leek Soup

It's amazing how just a handful of humble ingredients can be so easily transformed into this thoroughly satisfying and delicious soup. For a creamier version, stir in a bit of almond or other nut- or grain-based milk and heat through just before serving.

Tip Leeks need thorough and careful cleaning. To clean them, slice the leeks and immerse them in a bowl of cold water. Agitate them with your fingers. Lift the leeks out of the bowl and pour out the water and any sand or grit that has accumulated on the bottom of the bowl. Repeat several times until no more grit can be seen at the bottom of the bowl.

2 TABLESPOONS OLIVE OIL

3 LEEKS, THINLY SLICED AND
    THOROUGHLY CLEANED

2 CUPS CUBED YUKON GOLD
    POTATOES (1-INCH CUBES)

5 CUPS VEGETABLE STOCK

1 TEASPOON SEA SALT

½ TEASPOON FRESHLY GROUND
    BLACK PEPPER

3 TABLESPOONS CHOPPED
    FRESH CHIVES

1. In a large pot over medium-high heat, heat the olive oil until it shimmers. Add the leeks and cook until they soften, about 5 minutes. Add the potatoes, vegetable stock, salt, and pepper and cook until potatoes soften, about 10 minutes.

2. Transfer the soup to a blender or food processor, or use an immersion blender, and purée. Taste and adjust the seasonings. Serve hot, topped with chives.

Asian Noodle Soup

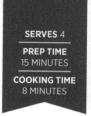
SERVES 4
PREP TIME
15 MINUTES
COOKING TIME
8 MINUTES

This soup is quick and simple to make, and most of the ingredients can be kept in the pantry so that you can have a steaming bowl of it any time you please. Sesame oil, chili oil, ginger, and star anise give this fragrant soup its distinctive Asian flavors.

2 TABLESPOONS OLIVE OIL

4 GREEN ONIONS (WHITE AND GREEN PARTS), JULIENNED

2 CARROTS, JULIENNED

1 TABLESPOON GRATED FRESH GINGER

3 GARLIC CLOVES, MINCED

6 CUPS VEGETABLE STOCK

1 STAR ANISE POD

6 OUNCES RICE NOODLES

1 TEASPOON SESAME OIL

½ TABLESPOON CHILI OIL

1. In a large pot, heat the olive oil until it shimmers. Add the green onions and carrots and cook until soft, about 4 minutes.

2. Add the ginger and garlic and cook until they are fragrant, about 30 seconds. Add the vegetable stock and anise pod and bring to a boil.

3. Add the rice noodles, sesame oil, and chili oil. Cook until the noodles soften, about 3 minutes. Remove the anise pod and serve immediately.

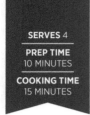

Creamy Mushroom Soup

The trick to the great mushroom flavor in this soup is dried porcini mushrooms, which you can find in the produce section. If you can't find dried porcinis, use any dried mushrooms. Soak them in hot stock for a couple of hours for best results.

5 CUPS VEGETABLE STOCK

ONE 1-OUNCE PACKAGE DRIED
    PORCINI MUSHROOMS

3 TABLESPOONS CORNSTARCH

½ CUP UNSWEETENED ALMOND MILK

2 TABLESPOONS OLIVE OIL

1 ONION, CHOPPED

2 CUPS SLICED CREMINI MUSHROOMS

3 GARLIC CLOVES, MINCED

1 TEASPOON DRIED THYME

SEA SALT

FRESHLY GROUND BLACK PEPPER

1. In a large bowl, combine the vegetable stock and dried mushrooms. Cover with plastic wrap and cut two 1-inch slits in the plastic. Microwave on high for 4 minutes. Allow the mushrooms to soak in the stock for 1 to 2 hours. Rinse the grit off the mushrooms and strain the grit out of the stock. Return the mushrooms to the stock.

2. In a small bowl, whisk together the cornstarch and almond milk until well combined. Set aside.

3. In a large soup pot, heat the olive oil over medium-high heat until it shimmers. Add the onion and mushrooms and cook until the vegetables soften, about 5 minutes. Add the garlic and cook until it is fragrant, about 30 seconds.

4. Add the stock-mushroom mixture, cornstarch mixture, and thyme. Cook, stirring occasionally, until the soup heats and thickens, about 10 minutes. Season with salt and pepper. Serve immediately.

Black Bean Soup

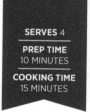

SERVES 4

PREP TIME
10 MINUTES

COOKING TIME
15 MINUTES

Using canned black beans ensures that this soup cooks quickly. If you purée the soup in a food processor or blender, be sure to protect your hand with a folded towel and allow steam to escape out the top.

2 TABLESPOONS OLIVE OIL

1 ONION, DICED

1 GREEN BELL PEPPER, DICED

1 CARROT, PEELED AND DICED

4 GARLIC CLOVES, MINCED

TWO 15-OUNCE CANS BLACK BEANS,
    DRAINED AND RINSED

2 CUPS VEGETABLE STOCK

¼ TEASPOON GROUND CUMIN

1 TEASPOON SEA SALT

¼ CUP CHOPPED CILANTRO,
    FOR GARNISH

1. In a large soup pot, heat the olive oil over medium-high heat until it shimmers. Add the onion, bell pepper, and carrot and cook until the vegetables soften, about 5 minutes. Add garlic and cook until it is fragrant, about 30 seconds.

2. Add the black beans, vegetable stock, cumin, and salt. Cook over medium-high heat, stirring occasionally, for about 10 minutes.

3. Remove from the heat. Using a potato masher, mash the beans lightly, leaving some chunks in the soup. For a smoother soup, process in a blender or food processor. Serve hot, garnished with cilantro.

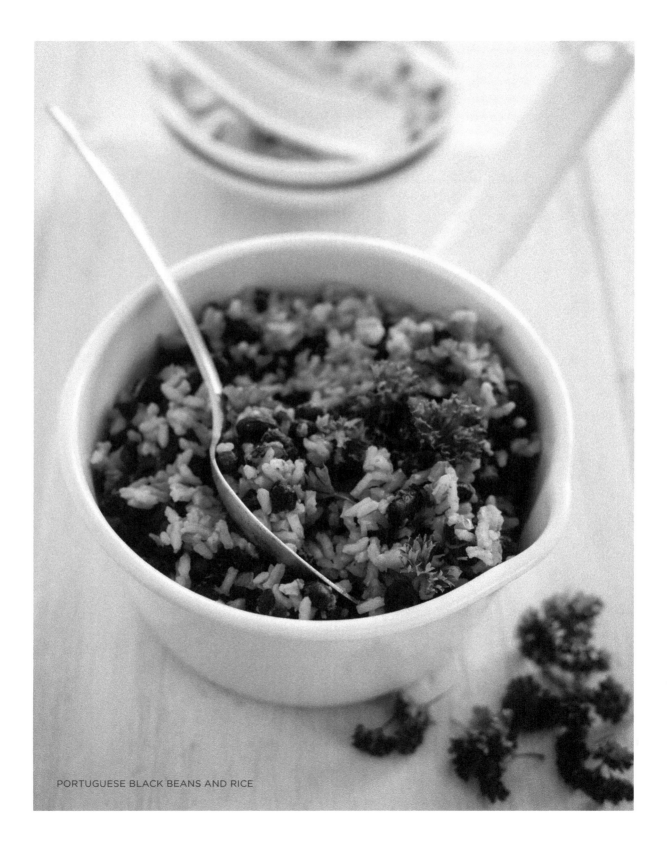

PORTUGUESE BLACK BEANS AND RICE

8

Beans and Grains

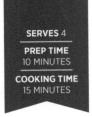
Quinoa Pilaf

Using quinoa in this pilaf is a nice variation on the more traditional rice pilaf. Plus, quinoa is loaded with protein and fiber, so along with a vegetable dish, it can make for a filling meal.

Tip Quinoa cooks quickly, but it also keeps well. You can make a large batch on the weekend and store it in an airtight container in the refrigerator for up to a week, reheating portions in the microwave as needed.

1 CUP QUINOA

2 CUPS VEGETABLE STOCK

¼ CUP PINE NUTS

2 TABLESPOONS OLIVE OIL

½ ONION, CHOPPED

⅓ CUP CHOPPED FRESH PARSLEY

SEA SALT

FRESHLY GROUND BLACK PEPPER

1. In a medium pot, bring the quinoa and vegetable stock to a boil over medium-high heat, stirring occasionally. Reduce to a simmer. Cover and cook until the quinoa is soft, about 15 minutes.

2. Meanwhile, heat a large sauté pan over medium-high heat. Add the pine nuts to the dry hot pan and toast, stirring frequently, until the nuts are fragrant, 2 to 3 minutes. Remove the pine nuts from the pan and set aside.

3. Add the olive oil to the same pan and heat until it shimmers. Add the onion and cook until soft, about 5 minutes.

4. When the quinoa is soft and all the liquid is absorbed, remove it from the heat and fluff it with a fork. Stir in the pine nuts, onion, and parsley. Season with salt and pepper. Serve hot.

Lemon and Thyme Couscous

SERVES 6

PREP TIME
5 MINUTES

COOKING TIME
10 MINUTES

Lemon and thyme are a classic aromatic pairing that lends delicious herbal and citrus flavor to this couscous. Serve it alongside garlicky sautéed vegetables for an easy lunch or to round out a meal of grilled vegetables and cool dips for a summer barbecue.

Tip This recipe is very versatile. Try substituting orange for the lemon, and oregano, mint, or basil for the thyme.

2¾ CUPS VEGETABLE STOCK

JUICE AND ZEST OF 1 LEMON

2 TABLESPOONS CHOPPED
   FRESH THYME

1½ CUPS COUSCOUS

¼ CUP CHOPPED FRESH PARSLEY

SEA SALT

FRESHLY GROUND BLACK PEPPER

1. In a medium pot, bring the vegetable stock, lemon juice, and thyme to a boil. Stir in the couscous, cover, and remove from the heat. Allow to sit, covered, until the couscous absorbs the liquid and softens, about 5 minutes. Fluff with a fork.

2. Stir in the lemon zest and parsley. Season with salt and pepper. Serve hot.

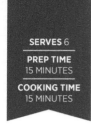
Mushroom Couscous

Because couscous cooks fast—it needs just 5 minutes of soaking in boiling liquid—this dish can be on the table in no time. Do note, however, that the dried mushrooms need to soak for at least an hour beforehand, so plan accordingly.

Tip While porcini are the most flavorful dried mushrooms, if you can't find them, you can substitute other dried mushrooms, such as shiitake or oyster, or substitute mushroom stock for the vegetable stock.

2¾ CUPS VEGETABLE STOCK

ONE 1-OUNCE PACKAGE DRIED
   PORCINI MUSHROOMS

1½ CUPS COUSCOUS

2 TABLESPOONS OLIVE OIL

½ ONION, CHOPPED

2 CUPS SLICED BUTTON MUSHROOMS

3 GARLIC CLOVES, MINCED

2 TEASPOONS FRESH THYME

SEA SALT

FRESHLY GROUND BLACK PEPPER

1. In a medium bowl, pour the vegetable stock over the porcini mushrooms. Cover and set aside for 1 to 2 hours.

2. Rinse the grit off the mushrooms and strain the grit out of the stock, then return the mushrooms to the stock.

3. In a medium pot, heat the vegetable stock with mushrooms over high heat until it boils. Add the couscous, stir, cover, and remove from the heat. Allow to sit until the couscous absorbs the liquid and softens, about 5 minutes.

4. Meanwhile, in a large sauté pan, heat the olive oil over medium-high heat until it shimmers. Add the onion and cook until soft, about 5 minutes. Add the button mushrooms and cook until soft, about 5 minutes. Add the garlic and cook until it is fragrant, about 30 seconds.

5. Fluff the couscous with a fork. Stir the mushroom mixture into the couscous. Add the thyme and season with salt and pepper. Serve immediately.

Fried Rice

SERVES 6

PREP TIME
10 MINUTES

COOKING TIME
15 MINUTES

Using precooked rice saves time in this recipe. Flavored with sesame oil, garlic, ginger, and soy sauce, it's a classic Asian side dish that goes well with Sweet and Sour Tempeh (page 122), General Tso's Tofu (page 140), or any Asian-style entrée.

Tip Making fried rice is a great way to use up leftover rice. For best results, use cold rice straight out of the refrigerator and rub between wet hands to separate the grains before adding them to the pan.

2 TABLESPOONS SESAME OIL

1 ONION, DICED

1 CARROT, DICED

1 CUP SUGAR SNAP PEAS

1 CUP SLICED SHIITAKE MUSHROOMS

2 GARLIC CLOVES, MINCED

1 TABLESPOON GRATED FRESH GINGER

¼ CUP SOY SAUCE

2 CUPS PREPARED RICE (BROWN OR WHITE)

3 GREEN ONIONS (WHITE AND GREEN PARTS), CHOPPED

1. In a large sauté pan or wok, heat the sesame oil until it shimmers. Add the onion and carrot. Cook until the vegetables soften, about 3 minutes.

2. Add the peas and mushrooms and cook, stirring frequently, until they soften, 5 to 7 minutes. Add the garlic and ginger and cook until they are fragrant, about 30 seconds.

3. Add the soy sauce and rice. Cook, stirring, until heated through. Stir in the green onions and serve immediately.

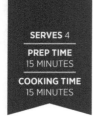

Curried Lentils

Curried lentils are a traditional Indian dish. Combined with brown rice, it's a meal full of protein, fiber, and lots of other nutrients. If you like your curry spicy, choose a spicy curry powder or add a dash of cayenne pepper.

Tip While you can use any type of lentils, golden lentils are especially good in this dish. If you don't want to use canned lentils, you can precook a batch of lentils on the weekend to use instead. You'll need about 4 cups of cooked lentils.

2 TABLESPOONS OLIVE OIL

1 ONION, DICED

2 CARROTS, DICED

2 CELERY STALKS, DICED

4 GARLIC CLOVES, MINCED

ONE 15-OUNCE CAN CHOPPED
    TOMATOES, INCLUDING JUICE

TWO 15-OUNCE CANS LENTILS,
    DRAINED AND RINSED

2 TEASPOONS CURRY POWDER

SEA SALT

FRESHLY GROUND BLACK PEPPER

2 TABLESPOONS CHOPPED CILANTRO

1. In a large pot, heat the olive oil over medium-high heat until it shimmers. Add the onion, carrots, and celery and cook until the vegetables soften, about 5 minutes.

2. Add the garlic and cook until it is fragrant, about 30 seconds. Add the tomatoes with juice, lentils, and curry powder and cook to combine the flavors, 9 to 10 minutes. Season with salt and pepper. Stir in the cilantro and serve immediately.

Spicy Picnic Beans

SERVES 6

PREP TIME
15 MINUTES

COOKING TIME
15 MINUTES

These zippy beans have a peppery heat because peppers are finely minced in a food processor before being combined with the beans. For extra spiciness, don't seed the jalapeño before mincing it. For less heat, remove the seeds and ribs of the chile before mincing.

1 JALAPEÑO, CUT INTO STRIPS

1 RED BELL PEPPER, CUT INTO STRIPS

1 GREEN BELL PEPPER, CUT INTO STRIPS

1 ONION, CHOPPED

5 GARLIC CLOVES, MINCED

TWO 15-OUNCE CANS PINTO BEANS, DRAINED AND RINSED

ONE 15-OUNCE CAN KIDNEY BEANS, DRAINED AND RINSED

ONE 15-OUNCE CAN CHICKPEAS, DRAINED AND RINSED

ONE 18-OUNCE BOTTLE BARBECUE SAUCE

½ TEASPOON CHIPOTLE POWDER

SEA SALT

FRESHLY GROUND BLACK PEPPER

1. In the bowl of a food processor, combine the jalapeño, bell peppers, onion, and garlic and blend for ten 1-second pulses, stopping halfway through to scrape down the sides of the bowl.

2. In a large pot, combine the processed mixture with the beans, barbecue sauce, and chipotle powder. Simmer over medium-high heat, stirring frequently to blend the flavors, about 15 minutes.

3. Season with salt and pepper. Serve hot. You can make this ahead of time and store it in a tightly sealed container for up to 3 days in the refrigerator. The flavors will blend and deepen as the beans rest.

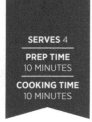
Chickpeas with Lemon and Spinach

This simple chickpea dish takes only a few minutes to make, but paired with cooked rice, baked sweet potatoes, or a basic pasta, it becomes a tasty and satisfying meal.

3 TABLESPOONS OLIVE OIL
ONE 15-OUNCE CAN CHICKPEAS,
    DRAINED AND RINSED
10 OUNCES BABY SPINACH

½ TEASPOON SEA SALT
JUICE AND ZEST OF 1 LEMON
FRESHLY GROUND BLACK PEPPER

1. In a large sauté pan, heat the olive oil over medium-high heat until it shimmers. Add the chickpeas and cook until they are heated through, about 5 minutes.

2. Add the spinach and stir just until it wilts, about 5 minutes. Add the salt, lemon juice, lemon zest, and pepper and stir to combine. Serve immediately.

Portuguese Black Beans and Rice

SERVES 4

PREP TIME
15 MINUTES

COOKING TIME
15 MINUTES

Chipotle chiles—smoked jalapeños usually sold canned in a rich adobo sauce—and smoked paprika add a robust heat to this delicious rice dish. You can find chipotle in adobo at the supermarket with the canned chiles.

2 TABLESPOONS OLIVE OIL

1 RED ONION, CHOPPED

2 BELL PEPPERS (RED, YELLOW, OR ORANGE), CHOPPED

4 GARLIC CLOVES, CHOPPED

3 CHIPOTLE CHILES IN ADOBO, CHOPPED

2 TOMATOES, CHOPPED, OR ONE 15-OUNCE CAN CHOPPED STEWED TOMATOES

ONE 15-OUNCE CAN BLACK BEANS, DRAINED AND RINSED

2 TABLESPOONS SMOKED PAPRIKA

1 TEASPOON GROUND CUMIN

1 TEASPOON FRESHLY GROUND BLACK PEPPER

4 CUPS PREPARED BROWN RICE

SEA SALT

1. In a large Dutch oven over medium-high heat, heat the olive oil until it shimmers. Add the onion and bell peppers and cook, stirring occasionally, until the vegetables soften, about 5 minutes. Add the garlic and cook until it is fragrant, about 30 seconds.

2. Add the chipotle chiles and tomatoes. Stir to scrape any browned bits off the bottom of the pan. Add the beans, paprika, cumin, and black pepper.

3. Turn down the heat to medium-low. Simmer, stirring frequently, about 5 minutes to allow the flavors to blend.

4. Stir in rice and cook to heat through. Season with salt and serve.

Brown Rice and Lentils

Using canned or precooked lentils, precooked brown rice, canned tomatoes, and a few herbs and spices, this recipe is perfect for a weeknight dinner. A crisp green salad or some steamed vegetables on the side are all you need to round out the meal.

Tip Canned lentils cook quickly, but if you prefer, feel free to substitute 4 cups of cooked dried lentils, which you can make ahead of time and keep in the refrigerator for up to a week.

2 TABLESPOONS OLIVE OIL

1 ONION, DICED

1 CARROT, DICED

1 CELERY STALK, DICED

TWO 15-OUNCE CANS LENTILS,
  DRAINED AND RINSED

ONE 15-OUNCE CAN DICED TOMATOES
  WITH JUICE

1 TABLESPOON DRIED ROSEMARY

1 TABLESPOON GARLIC POWDER

2 CUPS PREPARED BROWN RICE

SEA SALT

FRESHLY GROUND BLACK PEPPER

1. In a large pot, heat the olive oil over medium-high heat until it shimmers. Add the onion, carrot, and celery and cook until the vegetables soften, about 5 minutes.

2. Add the lentils, tomatoes, rosemary, and garlic powder. Lower the heat to medium-low and simmer to blend the flavors, 5 to 7 minutes.

3. Stir the rice into lentils and heat through, 2 to 3 minutes. Season with salt and pepper and serve immediately.

Cajun Red Beans and Rice

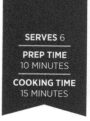
Cayenne pepper and Cajun seasoning add a pleasant heat to this rice-and-bean dish. It makes a great side, or you can serve large portions as a main dish with a fresh green salad as an accompaniment.

3 TABLESPOONS OLIVE OIL

1 ONION, CHOPPED

1 GREEN BELL PEPPER, CHOPPED

2 STALKS CELERY, CHOPPED

4 GARLIC CLOVES, MINCED

ONE 15-OUNCE CAN RED KIDNEY
    BEANS, DRAINED AND RINSED

½ TEASPOON CAYENNE PEPPER
   (OR TO TASTE)

1 TEASPOON DRIED THYME

1 TEASPOON CAJUN SEASONING

4 CUPS PREPARED BROWN RICE

SEA SALT

FRESHLY GROUND BLACK PEPPER

1. In a large pot, heat the olive oil over medium-high heat until it shimmers. Add the onion, bell pepper, and celery. Cook until the vegetables soften, stirring occasionally, about 5 minutes. Add the garlic and cook until it is fragrant, about 30 seconds.

2. Add the beans, cayenne, thyme, and Cajun seasoning. Turn down the heat to low and simmer, stirring occasionally, 5 to 7 minutes.

3. Stir the rice into the beans and heat through. Season with salt and black pepper and serve immediately.

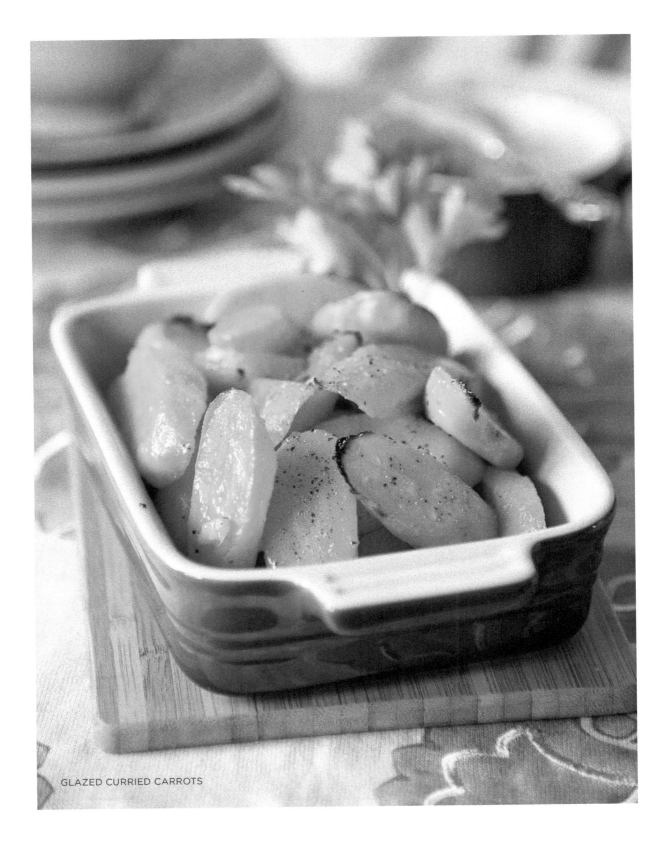

GLAZED CURRIED CARROTS

9

Vegetable Dishes

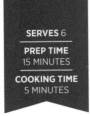

Green Beans Gremolata

Gremolata is a mixture of chopped herbs and citrus zest. This version uses oranges, which pair especially well with the green beans, although lemons would be a fine substitute.

Tip When zesting oranges, be careful not to get any of the white pith underneath, which will add bitterness.

1 POUND FRESH GREEN BEANS, TRIMMED, OR FROZEN OR CANNED GREEN BEANS

3 GARLIC CLOVES, MINCED

ZEST OF 2 ORANGES

3 TABLESPOONS MINCED FRESH PARSLEY

2 TABLESPOONS PINE NUTS

3 TABLESPOONS OLIVE OIL

SEA SALT

FRESHLY GROUND BLACK PEPPER

1. Fill a large pot about half full with water and bring to a boil over high heat. Add the green beans and cook for 2 to 3 minutes. Drain the beans in a colander and rinse with cold water to stop the cooking.

2. In a small bowl, mix the garlic, orange zest, and parsley.

3. In a large sauté pan over medium-high heat, toast the pine nuts in the dry, hot pan until they are fragrant, 2 to 3 minutes. Remove from the pan and set aside.

4. Heat the olive oil in the same pan until it shimmers. Add the beans and cook, stirring frequently, until heated through, about 2 minutes. Remove the pan from the heat and add the parsley mixture and pine nuts. Season with salt and pepper. Serve immediately.

Minted Peas

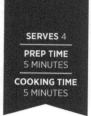
SERVES 4

PREP TIME
5 MINUTES

COOKING TIME
5 MINUTES

Mint and peas are a truly delightful combination. Using fresh spring peas is ideal, making this a perfectly seasonal springtime dish, but frozen peas are a totally acceptable substitute any time of year.

1 TABLESPOON OLIVE OIL

4 CUPS PEAS, FRESH OR FROZEN
(NOT CANNED)

½ TEASPOON SEA SALT

FRESHLY GROUND BLACK PEPPER

3 TABLESPOONS CHOPPED
FRESH MINT

In a large sauté pan, heat the olive oil over medium-high heat until hot. Add the peas and cook, about 5 minutes. Remove the pan from heat. Stir in the salt, season with pepper, and stir in the mint. Serve hot.

SERVES 4

PREP TIME
10 MINUTES

COOKING TIME
15 MINUTES

Sweet and Spicy Brussels Sprout Hash

Brussels sprouts are among those vegetables that many people say they don't like—until they taste a well-cooked version. This palate-pleasing dish balances the bitterness of Brussels sprouts with sweet maple syrup, acidic cider vinegar, and spicy Sriracha. Even avowed Brussels sprout haters will find it irresistible.

Tip Some supermarkets now carry sliced Brussels sprouts, which will save you tons of prep time. Look for them in the bagged salad section. If you can't find them, you can also use the slicing attachment on a food processor to slice a lot of Brussels sprouts quickly.

3 TABLESPOONS OLIVE OIL

2 SHALLOTS, THINLY SLICED

1½ POUNDS BRUSSELS SPROUTS,
    TRIMMED AND CUT INTO
    THIN SLICES

3 TABLESPOONS APPLE
    CIDER VINEGAR

1 TABLESPOON PURE MAPLE SYRUP

½ TEASPOON SRIRACHA SAUCE (OR
    TO TASTE)

SEA SALT

FRESHLY GROUND BLACK PEPPER

1. In a large sauté pan, heat the olive oil over medium-high heat until it shimmers. Add the shallots and Brussels sprouts and cook, stirring frequently, until the vegetables soften and begin to turn golden brown, about 10 minutes. Stir in the vinegar, using a spoon to scrape any browned bits from the bottom of the pan. Stir in the maple syrup and Sriracha.

2. Simmer, stirring frequently, until the liquid reduces, 3 to 5 minutes. Season with salt and pepper and serve immediately.

Glazed Curried Carrots

Coated with a sweet-spicy sauce of curry and maple syrup, these just might beat your mom's classic version as your favorite glazed carrot dish. Slice the carrots thinly so they will cook quickly, and simmer them gently with the maple syrup and curry until the sauce is reduced to a delicious glaze.

1 POUND CARROTS, PEELED AND
    THINLY SLICED
2 TABLESPOONS OLIVE OIL
2 TABLESPOONS CURRY POWDER

2 TABLESPOONS PURE MAPLE SYRUP
JUICE OF ½ LEMON
SEA SALT
FRESHLY GROUND BLACK PEPPER

1. Place the carrots in a large pot and cover with water. Cook on medium-high heat until tender, about 10 minutes. Drain the carrots and return them to the pan over medium-low heat.

2. Stir in the olive oil, curry powder, maple syrup, and lemon juice. Cook, stirring constantly, until the liquid reduces, about 5 minutes. Season with salt and pepper and serve immediately.

Pepper Medley

Bell peppers, garlic, and basil make for a classic Italian flavor profile. If you like, you can replace red wine vinegar with white wine vinegar.

3 TABLESPOONS OLIVE OIL

1 RED BELL PEPPER, SLICED

1 ORANGE BELL PEPPER, SLICED

1 YELLOW BELL PEPPER, SLICED

1 GREEN BELL PEPPER, SLICED

2 GARLIC CLOVES, MINCED

3 TABLESPOONS RED WINE VINEGAR

SEA SALT

FRESHLY GROUND BLACK PEPPER

2 TABLESPOONS CHOPPED
   FRESH BASIL

1. In a large sauté pan, heat the olive oil over medium-high heat until it shimmers. Add the bell peppers and cook, stirring frequently, until softened, 7 to 10 minutes. Add the garlic and cook until it is fragrant, about 30 seconds. Add the vinegar, using a spoon to scrape any browned bits off the bottom of the pan.

2. Simmer until the vinegar reduces, 2 to 3 minutes. Season with salt and pepper. Stir in the basil and serve immediately.

Garlicky Red Wine Mushrooms

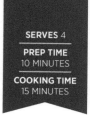

SERVES 4

PREP TIME
10 MINUTES

COOKING TIME
15 MINUTES

This recipe works equally well with button or cremini mushrooms or more exotic wild mushrooms like porcini or chanterelles. Wild mushrooms can be pricey, so for a flavorful yet still economical version, try a mix of regular supermarket mushrooms and a more exotic type.

Tip Avoid waterlogging mushrooms by cleaning them with a slightly damp paper towel or mushroom brush instead of rinsing them.

3 TABLESPOONS OLIVE OIL

2 CUPS SLICED MUSHROOMS

3 GARLIC CLOVES, MINCED

½ CUP RED WINE

1 TABLESPOON DRIED THYME

SEA SALT

FRESHLY GROUND BLACK PEPPER

1. In a large sauté pan, heat the olive oil over medium-high heat until it shimmers. Add the mushrooms and allow to sit, untouched, until they release their liquid and begin to brown, about 5 minutes. Stir the mushrooms occasionally, cooking until softened and golden brown, about 5 minutes more. Add the garlic and cook until it is fragrant, about 30 seconds. Add the red wine and thyme, using a wooden spoon to scrape any browned bits off the bottom of the pan.

2. Lower the heat to medium and cook until the wine reduces, 4 to 5 minutes. Season with salt and pepper and serve immediately.

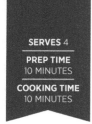
Sautéed Citrus Spinach

Spinach cooks fast, making this a quick and easy side dish, and the versatile flavors of orange and garlic will complement many different cuisines. If you prefer, you can use lemon zest and juice instead of orange. For a little heat, toss in a pinch of red pepper flakes along with the salt and pepper.

2 TABLESPOONS OLIVE OIL

1 SHALLOT, CHOPPED

2 GARLIC CLOVES, MINCED

10 OUNCES BABY SPINACH

ZEST AND JUICE OF 1 ORANGE

SEA SALT

FRESHLY GROUND BLACK PEPPER

1. In a large sauté pan, heat the olive oil over medium-high heat until it shimmers. Add the shallot and cook until soft, about 3 minutes. Add the garlic and cook until it is fragrant, about 30 seconds.

2. Add the spinach, orange juice, and orange zest. Cook, stirring, until the spinach wilts, 2 to 3 minutes. Season with salt and pepper. Serve warm.

Lemon Broccoli Rabe

SERVES 4

PREP TIME
10 MINUTES

COOKING TIME
10 MINUTES

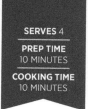

Broccoli rabe—which looks like a leafier version of broccoli with larger leaves, longer and thinner stems, and smaller florets—is actually a member of the turnip family. Like turnip or mustard greens, the entire plant (including the buds, leaves, and stems) is edible. The flavor is slightly bitter, making it a good partner for tart lemon.

8 CUPS WATER

SEA SALT

2 BUNCHES BROCCOLI RABE, CHOPPED

3 TABLESPOONS OLIVE OIL

3 GARLIC CLOVES, MINCED

PINCH OF CAYENNE PEPPER

ZEST OF 1 LEMON

FRESHLY GROUND BLACK PEPPER

1. In a large pot, bring 8 cups of the water to a boil. Add a pinch of salt and the broccoli rabe. Cook until the broccoli rabe is slightly softened, about 2 minutes. Drain.

2. In a large sauté pan, heat the olive oil over medium-high heat until it shimmers. Add the garlic and cook until it is fragrant, about 30 seconds. Stir in the broccoli rabe, cayenne, and lemon zest. Season with salt and black pepper. Serve immediately.

Spicy Swiss Chard

This recipe uses both the leaves and the stems of the chard, cooking them separately. If you use a brightly colored chard—it comes in red, golden, and rainbow in addition to the standard green—the stems will add a bright pop of color to the finished dish.

2 TABLESPOONS OLIVE OIL

1 ONION, CHOPPED

2 BUNCHES SWISS CHARD, STEMS AND
    LEAVES SEPARATED, CHOPPED

3 GARLIC CLOVES, MINCED

½ TEASPOON RED PEPPER FLAKES
    (OR TO TASTE)

JUICE OF ½ LEMON, OR 2 TEASPOONS
    PREPARED LEMON JUICE

SEA SALT

1. In a large pot, heat the olive oil over medium-high heat until it shimmers. Add the onion and chard stems and cook until soft, about 5 minutes.

2. Add the chard leaves and cook until they wilt, about 1 minute. Stir in the garlic and pepper flakes. Cover and cook until tender, 4 to 5 minutes. Stir in the lemon juice. Season with salt and serve immediately.

Red Peppers and Kale

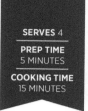

Dark, leafy greens like kale are full of heart-healthy compounds. Bright red peppers are loaded with vitamin C. This sauté offers an ample portion of both, making it as good for you as it is delicious.

2 BUNCHES KALE, STALKS REMOVED
    AND CUT INTO SMALL PIECES
3 TABLESPOONS OLIVE OIL
½ ONION, CHOPPED
2 RED BELL PEPPERS, CUT INTO STRIPS

3 GARLIC CLOVES, MINCED
¼ TEASPOON RED PEPPER FLAKES
SEA SALT
FRESHLY GROUND BLACK PEPPER

1. In steamer basket in a pan, steam the kale until it softens, 5 to 10 minutes. Remove from the heat and set aside.

2. Meanwhile, in a sauté pan, heat the olive oil over medium-high heat until it shimmers. Add the onion and bell peppers and cook until soft, about 5 minutes. Add the garlic and cook until it is fragrant, about 30 seconds. Remove from the heat and stir in the kale and red pepper flakes. Season with salt and black pepper and serve immediately.

Mashed Cauliflower with Roasted Garlic

If you're watching your carb intake and miss mashed potatoes, pine no more. This is a lower-carb version of that beloved dish. The roasted garlic adds a rich sweetness to the purée for a flavor so deeply satisfying you'll hardly notice that cauliflower has replaced the potatoes.

Tip To make your own roasted garlic, preheat the oven to 400°F. With a sharp knife, cut about ½ inch off the top of a bulb of garlic so that the individual cloves are exposed. Place this on a square of aluminum foil and drizzle with a tablespoon or two of olive oil. Wrap the foil loosely around the garlic so that it is sealed but there is room inside for heat to circulate. Roast in the preheated oven for about 45 minutes, until the cloves are soft and golden brown.

2 HEADS CAULIFLOWER, CUT INTO
    SMALL FLORETS
1 TABLESPOON OLIVE OIL
8 JARRED ROASTED GARLIC CLOVES
2 TEASPOONS CHOPPED FRESH
    ROSEMARY

SEA SALT
FRESHLY GROUND BLACK PEPPER
1 TABLESPOON CHOPPED
    FRESH CHIVES

1. Add cauliflower florets to a large pot and cover with water. Cover and bring to a boil over high heat. Cook until tender, 8 to 10 minutes, then drain.

2. In a blender or food processor, combine the cauliflower, olive oil, garlic, and rosemary and process until smooth. Season with salt and pepper. Stir in the chives and serve hot.

Steamed Broccoli with Walnut Pesto

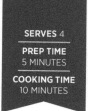

SERVES 4

PREP TIME
5 MINUTES

COOKING TIME
10 MINUTES

Basic steamed broccoli gets a welcome makeover with the addition of a rich, nutty walnut pesto that's easy to whip up. For a mellower pesto, toast the walnuts before adding them to the other pesto ingredients in the food processor.

Tip To toast walnuts, heat a sauté pan over medium-high heat. Add the walnuts and cook, stirring frequently, for about 3 minutes, until the nuts become fragrant and just start to brown.

1 POUND BROCCOLI FLORETS

2 CUPS CHOPPED FRESH BASIL

¼ CUP OLIVE OIL

4 GARLIC CLOVES

½ CUP WALNUTS

PINCH OF CAYENNE PEPPER

1. Put the broccoli in a large pot and cover with water. Bring to a simmer over medium-high heat and cook until the broccoli is tender, about 5 minutes.

2. Meanwhile, in a food processor, combine the basil, olive oil, garlic, walnuts, and cayenne and blend for ten 1-second pulses, scraping down the bowl halfway through processing.

3. Drain the broccoli and return to the pan. Toss with the pesto. Serve immediately.

Roasted Asparagus with Balsamic Reduction

Roasting asparagus brings out its sweet notes and the tips get slightly brown and crispy, making them especially tasty. Meyer lemons are sweeter and juicier than common lemons. Their flavor pairs beautifully with the asparagus here.

Tip The fastest way to trim asparagus is to bend it near the root end until it snaps. The spears will naturally break just where the woody root end stops and the tender, edible part of the shoot begins.

1½ POUNDS ASPARAGUS, TRIMMED
2 TABLESPOONS OLIVE OIL
½ TEASPOON SEA SALT

¼ TEASPOON FRESHLY GROUND
BLACK PEPPER
⅓ CUP BALSAMIC VINEGAR
JUICE AND ZEST OF 1 MEYER LEMON

1. Preheat the oven to 375°F. On a large rimmed baking sheet, toss the asparagus with the olive oil, salt, and pepper and then spread the asparagus out into a single layer. Roast for 20 to 25 minutes, stirring once, until tender and beginning to brown.

2. While the asparagus is roasting, put the vinegar in a small saucepan and bring it to a boil over medium-high heat. Turn down the heat to low and simmer until reduced to a thick syrup, about 8 minutes.

3. When the asparagus is roasted, remove the baking sheet from the oven. Add the lemon juice and zest and toss to coat. Transfer to a serving platter and drizzle the balsamic reduction over the top. Serve immediately.

Tempura Vegetables with Ponzu-Style Sauce

SERVES 4

PREP TIME
15 MINUTES

COOKING TIME
10 MINUTES

These crispy morsels are a delicious way to use up a random assortment of veggies in your fridge. In fact, practically any vegetable will work well as long as it's not too soft or juicy. Root vegetables, onions, or florets of broccoli or cauliflower work especially well.

Tip Ponzu sauce is traditionally made with the juice of the yuzu fruit, an Asian citrus with a flavor that resembles a sweet grapefruit. Here we use lemon juice in its place, but you could substitute orange, tangerine, or Meyer lemon if you like.

FOR THE SAUCE
½ CUP SOY SAUCE
¼ CUP RICE WINE VINEGAR
¼ CUP LEMON JUICE

FOR THE TEMPURA
1 QUART PEANUT OIL
1 CUP CORNSTARCH
1 CUP ALL-PURPOSE FLOUR
2 CUPS CHILLED CLUB SODA

6 CUPS ASSORTED VEGETABLES, PEELED AND CUT INTO STICKS OR WEDGES (CARROTS, BROCCOLI, CAULIFLOWER, BUTTON MUSHROOMS, ONION RINGS, OR SUMMER OR WINTER SQUASH)
SEA SALT

1. Heat the peanut oil to 350°F in a deep, wide saucepan.

2. In a small bowl, make the sauce by stirring together the soy sauce, vinegar, and lemon juice.

3. In a large bowl, stir together the cornstarch and flour. Add the club soda and stir to combine, but do not overmix.

4. Dunk one vegetable piece at a time into the flour mixture, letting the excess drip back into the bowl. Drop into the hot oil. Repeat with several pieces of vegetable without crowding the pan. Cook, turning occasionally, until the batter turns golden brown and crisp all over, about 2 minutes. Transfer the vegetables as they are cooked to a paper towel–lined plate. Sprinkle each batch with a bit of salt as it comes out of the oil. Repeat until all of the vegetables have been cooked. Serve immediately drizzled with the sauce.

Braised Eggplant

Here, silky eggplant is coated with a rich, thick, and spicy sauce. Serve this dish over steamed rice—either white or brown—so that you don't waste any of the delicious sauce. You can use either long, thin Asian eggplants or the larger plump, oval-shaped European ones in this dish.

Tip Shaoxing wine and fermented black bean chili paste can both be found in Asian grocery stores or in the Asian foods aisle in many supermarkets.

3 POUNDS EGGPLANT, CUT INTO
    2-INCH PIECES

2 TEASPOONS RICE VINEGAR

¾ CUP SHAOXING WINE, DRY SHERRY,
    OR DRY WHITE WINE

1 TABLESPOON CORNSTARCH

3 TABLESPOONS SOY SAUCE

2 TABLESPOONS BROWN SUGAR

1 TABLESPOON FERMENTED
    BLACK BEAN CHILI PASTE

1 TABLESPOON TOASTED SESAME OIL

2 TABLESPOONS VEGETABLE OIL

6 GARLIC CLOVES, 2 SMASHED WITH
    THE SIDE OF A KNIFE AND
    4 THINLY SLICED

2 GREEN ONIONS (WHITE AND GREEN
    PARTS), THINLY SLICED

¼ CUP CHOPPED CILANTRO, FOR
    GARNISH

1. In a steamer basket set over boiling water, steam the eggplant until it is tender, about 10 minutes.

2. Meanwhile, make the sauce by stirring together the vinegar, wine, and cornstarch in a small bowl. Stir in the soy sauce, brown sugar, chili paste, and sesame oil.

3. In a large, heavy skillet over medium-high heat, heat the vegetable oil. When the oil is hot, add the 2 whole garlic cloves. Lower the heat to medium and cook, stirring and turning the garlic cloves, until they turn golden brown, about 5 minutes. Remove and discard the garlic cloves.

4. Heat the pan over high heat until the oil is very hot and nearly smoking. Add the sliced garlic and green onions and cook, stirring, for 1 minute. Give the sauce mixture a quick stir and then add it to the skillet. Add the eggplant and bring the mixture to a boil. Reduce the heat to low and simmer, stirring occasionally, until the sauce becomes thick and glossy, about 5 minutes. Serve immediately garnished with the chopped cilantro.

NOTES

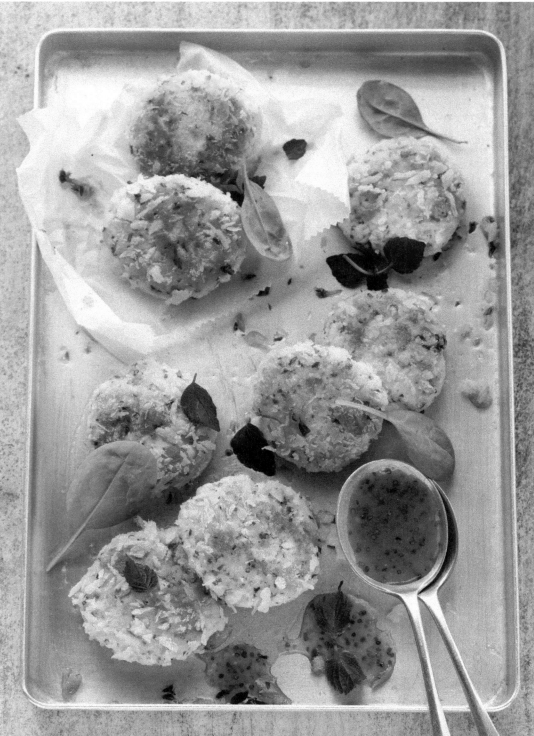

TOFU CAKES

10

Main Courses

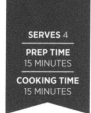

Spicy Nut-Butter Noodles

Use any nut butter you like with these noodles, such as peanut butter, cashew butter, or almond butter. While the recipe calls for this to be served hot, you can also serve it chilled as a salad.

Tip If you're allergic to peanuts and/or tree nuts, tahini (sesame seed paste) is a great alternative to use here. Look for it in the health food or ethnic food aisle of your supermarket, at natural foods stores, or at Middle Eastern markets.

1 PACKAGE SOBA NOODLES

½ CUP VEGETABLE STOCK

1 TABLESPOON MINCED FRESH GINGER

2 GARLIC CLOVES, MINCED

¼ CUP SOY SAUCE

¼ CUP PEANUT BUTTER OR OTHER
    NUT BUTTER

1 TEASPOON SRIRACHA OR CHILI
    PASTE

4 GREEN ONIONS (WHITE AND GREEN
    PARTS), CHOPPED

CHOPPED PEANUTS (OPTIONAL)

1. Prepare the soba noodles according to package directions. Drain and set aside.

2. In a small saucepan, combine the vegetable stock, ginger, garlic, soy sauce, peanut butter, and Sriracha, over medium-high heat, stirring until the peanut butter is melted and the sauce is heated through.

3. Toss the sauce with the hot noodles. Top with chopped green onions and peanuts, if using. Serve immediately.

Rigatoni with Roasted Tomatoes and Arugula

SERVES 4

PREP TIME
15 MINUTES

COOKING TIME
20 MINUTES

The rigatoni in this recipe combines with roasted vegetables, green olives, and arugula to create a classically delicious taste. If you like, you can replace the pasta with bow tie pasta, or replace the arugula with baby spinach.

1 PINT CHERRY TOMATOES

3 SHALLOTS, THINLY SLICED

SEA SALT

FRESHLY GROUND BLACK PEPPER

3 TABLESPOONS EXTRA VIRGIN
    OLIVE OIL

ONE 9-OUNCE BOX RIGATONI PASTA

3 CLOVES GARLIC, MINCED

3 TABLESPOONS RED WINE VINEGAR

4 OUNCES GREEN OLIVES, HALVED

¼ TEASPOON RED PEPPER FLAKES

2 CUPS BABY ARUGULA

1. Preheat the oven to 400°F.

2. Bring a large pot of water to boil over high heat.

3. In a large ovenproof sauté pan, place cherry tomatoes and shallots in a single layer. Season to taste with sea salt and black pepper and drizzle with the olive oil. Put the pan in the preheated oven and cook for 20 minutes, until the tomatoes and shallots are soft.

4. Meanwhile, add the rigatoni to the boiling water. Cook according to the package directions until the pasta is al dente, nine to twelve minutes. Drain the pasta.

5. When the tomatoes and shallots are done roasting, move the pan to the stovetop and turn the stove on medium-high. Be careful not to touch the handle of the pan without a potholder.

6. Add the garlic to the pan and cook, stirring constantly, until it is fragrant, about 30 seconds.

7. Add the red wine vinegar and olives to the pan, using the side of the spoon to scrape any browned bits from the bottom of the pan. Bring to a simmer and stir in the red pepper flakes.

8. Toss the vegetables with the pasta, stirring in the arugula, which will wilt slightly from the heat. Serve immediately.

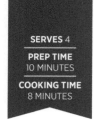

SERVES 4

PREP TIME
10 MINUTES

COOKING TIME
8 MINUTES

Sweet and Sour Tempeh

This popular Chinese-American dish is usually made with pork, but the tempeh here makes for a fine substitute coated with the flavorful sauce. Pineapple juice adds the sweetness, which is perfectly balanced by the sour rice vinegar. Serve this dish with Fried Rice (page 93) or plain steamed rice. You can also stir in chunks of pineapple for a brighter flavor.

1 CUP PINEAPPLE JUICE

1 TABLESPOON UNSEASONED
   RICE VINEGAR

1 TABLESPOON SOY SAUCE

1 TABLESPOON CORNSTARCH

2 TABLESPOONS COCONUT OIL

1 POUND TEMPEH, CUT INTO THIN STRIPS

6 GREEN ONIONS (WHITE AND GREEN
   PARTS), CUT INTO STRIPS

1 GREEN BELL PEPPER, DICED

4 GARLIC CLOVES, MINCED

2 CUPS PREPARED BROWN OR
   WHITE RICE

1. In a small bowl, whisk together the pineapple juice, rice vinegar, soy sauce, and cornstarch and set aside.

2. In a wok or large sauté pan, heat the coconut oil over medium-high heat until it shimmers. Add the tempeh, green onions, and bell pepper and cook until vegetables soften, about 5 minutes.

3. Add the garlic and cook until it is fragrant, about 30 seconds. Add the sauce and cook until it thickens, about 3 minutes. Serve over rice.

Fried Seitan Fingers

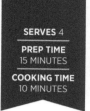

SERVES 4

PREP TIME
15 MINUTES

COOKING TIME
10 MINUTES

Strips of seitan are seasoned with classic Southern spices and then quickly fried to a crispy golden brown for a dish that is loved by adults and children alike. Serve them alongside Mashed Cauliflower with Roasted Garlic (page 112) and steamed vegetables for a family-friendly meal.

1 CUP ALL-PURPOSE FLOUR

1 TEASPOON GARLIC POWDER

1 TEASPOON ONION POWDER

PINCH OF CAYENNE PEPPER

1 TEASPOON DRIED THYME

½ TEASPOON SEA SALT

½ TEASPOON FRESHLY GROUND
    BLACK PEPPER

1 CUP SOY MILK

1 TABLESPOON LEMON JUICE

2 TABLESPOONS BAKING POWDER

2 TABLESPOONS OLIVE OIL

8 OUNCES SEITAN, CUT INTO
    ½-INCH-THICK "FINGERS"

1. In a shallow dish, combine the flour, garlic powder, onion powder, cayenne, thyme, salt, and black pepper, whisking to mix thoroughly. In another shallow dish, whisk together the soy milk, lemon juice, and baking powder.

2. In a large sauté pan, heat the olive oil over medium-high heat until it shimmers. Dip each piece of seitan in the flour mixture, tapping off any excess flour. Next, dip the seitan in the soy milk mixture and then back in the flour mixture.

3. Fry until golden brown on each side, 3 to 4 minutes per side. Blot on paper towels before serving.

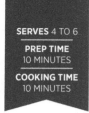
Lettuce Wraps with Spicy Tofu

Crunchy-yet-tender lettuce leaves make a great wrapper for chunks of tofu stir-fried with vegetables and ginger and seasoned with soy sauce and Sriracha. Buy premade dipping sauces, such as peanut sauce and sweet chili garlic sauce, as accompaniments.

Tip Butter lettuce has big, tender leaves that are perfect for holding all types of fillings. Be sure to dry the lettuce thoroughly after washing so the rolls won't be watered down.

2 TABLESPOONS COCONUT OIL
1 ONION, CHOPPED
1 CARROT, CHOPPED
1 TABLESPOON GRATED FRESH GINGER
3 GARLIC CLOVES, MINCED

1 POUND CRUMBLED EXTRA-FIRM TOFU
¼ CUP SOY SAUCE
1 TEASPOON SRIRACHA SAUCE
16 BUTTER LETTUCE LEAVES
1 CUP PREPARED PEANUT SAUCE

1. In a large sauté pan, heat the coconut oil over medium-high heat. Add the onion and carrot and cook until the vegetables soften, 5 to 7 minutes. Add the ginger and garlic and cook until they are fragrant, about 30 seconds.

2. Add the tofu and cook for another 4 minutes, breaking up the tofu with a spoon as you cook it. Add the soy sauce and Sriracha and cook for 1 or 2 minutes more, until heated through.

3. Serve with lettuce and peanut sauce, allowing diners to wrap the filling in lettuce leaves and dip finished wraps in the peanut sauce.

Tofu Cakes

SERVES 4
PREP TIME
15 MINUTES
COOKING TIME
15 MINUTES

Serve these flavorful tofu-and-vegetable patties with a side of steamed vegetables or oven-baked sweet potato fries—or, for a fun twist, make them a little larger and dish them up on hamburger buns with your favorite burger fixings.

1 POUND EXTRA-FIRM TOFU, CRUMBLED

2 CARROTS, PEELED AND GRATED

6 GREEN ONIONS (WHITE AND GREEN PARTS), DICED

4 GARLIC CLOVES, MINCED

¼ CUP CHOPPED CILANTRO

¼ CUP CHOPPED FRESH PARSLEY

1 TEASPOON SEA SALT

½ TEASPOON FRESHLY GROUND BLACK PEPPER

1½ CUPS BREAD CRUMBS

2 CUPS ALL-PURPOSE FLOUR

2 CUPS UNSWEETENED SOY MILK

¼ CUP OLIVE OIL

1. Line a baking sheet with parchment paper. In a large bowl, mash the tofu with a fork. Add the carrots, green onions, garlic, cilantro, parsley, salt, and pepper and stir carefully to combine. Place the bread crumbs, flour, and soy milk each in a shallow dish.

2. Working with about ⅓ cup at a time, shape the tofu mixture into patties. Dip each patty in the flour, tapping off any excess flour. Next, dip them in the soy milk and finally the bread crumbs. Set each patty on the baking sheet. Chill the prepared patties for 30 minutes.

3. In a large sauté pan or griddle, heat half the olive oil over medium-high heat until it shimmers. Fry the patties, cooking until golden, about 4 minutes per side, adding the remaining olive oil as needed. Serve hot.

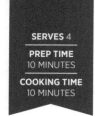
Tofu and Mushrooms

Tofu and mushrooms are seasoned with a sesame-ginger soy sauce and cook up in a flash under the broiler. Try them alongside Fried Rice (page 93), sesame-seasoned Asian noodles, or plain steamed rice for a healthy meal.

4 GARLIC CLOVES, MINCED

1 TABLESPOON GRATED FRESH GINGER

½ CUP SOY SAUCE

½ TEASPOON CHILI OIL

1 TABLESPOON SESAME OIL

1 POUND EXTRA-FIRM TOFU, CUT INTO
    BITE-SIZE PIECES

1 POUND SHIITAKE
    MUSHROOMS, CHOPPED

4 GREEN ONIONS (WHITE AND GREEN
    PARTS), CUT INTO STRIPS

¼ CUP CHOPPED CILANTRO

2 TABLESPOONS SESAME SEEDS

1. Heat the broiler to high. In a small bowl, whisk together the garlic, ginger, soy sauce, chili oil, and sesame oil.

2. Put the tofu and mushrooms in a large baking dish. Pour the soy-sauce mixture over the top. Place under the broiler and cook until the sauce bubbles, about 10 minutes. Sprinkle with the green onions, cilantro, and sesame seeds and serve hot.

Grilled Pesto Tofu

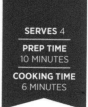
This quick and brightly flavored pesto contains nutritional yeast, which adds a savory flavor similar to the one traditionally contributed by Parmesan cheese. For an Italian-themed meal, serve this dish with fresh pasta and a fennel and radicchio salad with a simple vinaigrette.

Tip Pesto freezes surprisingly well. Make a large batch and freeze it in small portions using an ice cube tray. Once frozen, transfer the cubes to a freezer-safe plastic bag or other container. Add a cube to sauces or other dishes any time you want a hit of fresh Italian flavor.

1½ CUPS FRESH BASIL

⅓ CUP OLIVE OIL

1 CUP PINE NUTS

5 GARLIC CLOVES

⅓ CUP NUTRITIONAL YEAST

½ TEASPOON SEA SALT

½ TEASPOON FRESHLY GROUND
    BLACK PEPPER

1 POUND EXTRA-FIRM TOFU,
    DRAINED AND BLOTTED DRY
    ON A PAPER TOWEL

3 TABLESPOONS OLIVE OIL

1. Heat a grill to medium-high.

2. In the bowl of a food processer, combine the basil, ⅓ cup olive oil, pine nuts, garlic, nutritional yeast, salt, and pepper. Blend for ten 1-second pulses, scraping sides of bowl halfway through. Set aside.

3. Cut the tofu into four equal slices. Brush each with the olive oil and season lightly with salt and pepper. Grill for 2 to 3 minutes per side, until the tofu has grill marks and heats through. Serve hot, topped with pesto.

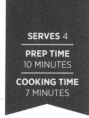
Orange and Soy Tofu

The classic Asian flavors of this dish go well with the Fried Rice recipe in this book (page 93) or steamed rice. Add a little Sriracha or a pinch of red pepper flakes for some heat.

¼ CUP SOY SAUCE

½ CUP ORANGE JUICE

1 TABLESPOON UNSEASONED
RICE VINEGAR

1 TEASPOON GRATED FRESH GINGER

1 TEASPOON CORNSTARCH

2 TABLESPOONS OLIVE OIL

3 GARLIC CLOVES, MINCED

1 POUND EXTRA-FIRM TOFU,
DRAINED, DRIED, AND CUT
INTO 1-INCH CUBES

1. In a small bowl, whisk together the soy sauce, orange juice, vinegar, ginger, and cornstarch. Set aside.

2. In a sauté pan, heat the olive oil over medium-high heat until it shimmers. Add the garlic and cook until it is fragrant, about 30 seconds. Add the tofu and cook, stirring frequently, until the tofu begins to brown, 3 to 4 minutes. Whisk the sauce one more time and add it to the tofu. Simmer until the sauce thickens and coats the tofu, about 3 minutes. Serve hot.

Naked Burritos

This recipe allows you to make the best part of the burritos—the inside. To serve, place all the ingredients on the table and allow diners to fill bowls with their favorites. You can use prepared guacamole or make your own using the Jicama and Guacamole recipe in this book (page 40).

TWO 15-OUNCE CANS BLACK BEANS,
    DRAINED AND RINSED
4 CUPS PREPARED WHITE OR
    BROWN RICE
ONE 15-OUNCE CAN SLICED BLACK
    OLIVES, DRAINED
1 TOMATO, CHOPPED

½ CUP CHOPPED CILANTRO
¼ CUP CHOPPED GREEN ONIONS
    (WHITE AND GREEN PARTS)
JUICE OF 2 TO 3 LIMES
1 CUP GUACAMOLE
1 CUP PREPARED SALSA
TORTILLA CHIPS, FOR SERVING

1. In a microwave-safe dish, heat the black beans until hot, 3 to 4 minutes. Set aside.

2. Heat the rice according to package directions. Divide the rice and beans evenly among four to six bowls. Layer with olives, tomato, cilantro, and green onions. Squeeze the juice of ½ lime over the top of each bowl and stir to combine. Top with guacamole, salsa, and crushed tortilla chips. Serve immediately.

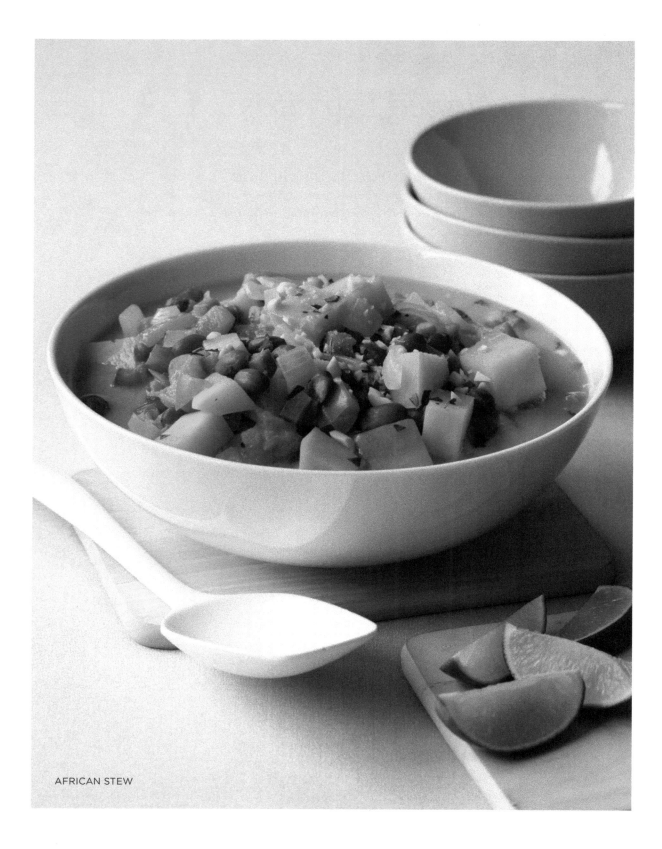

AFRICAN STEW

11

International Cuisine

Thai Spring Rolls

Filled with crunchy vegetables, chewy rice noodles, and fresh herbs, these rice paper–wrapped rolls are like a handheld salad. Make the rolls one at a time so the wrappers are less likely to tear. Once you get the hang of it, rolling them up is a cinch. You can find the wrappers in the Asian section of any supermarket.

1 CUP BEAN THREAD NOODLES

½ CUP BEAN SPROUTS

1 CUP SHREDDED CABBAGE

5 GREEN ONIONS (WHITE AND GREEN PARTS), CHOPPED

¼ CUP CHOPPED CILANTRO

1 CARROT, JULIENNED

1 TABLESPOON LIME JUICE

1 TABLESPOON SOY SAUCE

1 PACKAGE SPRING ROLL WRAPPERS

1. Put the bean thread noodles in a bowl of hot water and soak until soft, about 15 minutes. Drain the noodles and let cool to room temperature.

2. In a separate small bowl, combine the noodles, bean sprouts, cabbage, green onions, cilantro, carrot, lime juice, and soy sauce.

3. Fill another bowl with hot water. Working with one wrapper at a time, submerge the wrapper in hot water for about 15 seconds to soften and then lay on a piece of parchment paper. Spoon 2 tablespoons of the vegetable mixture onto each wrapper and roll it carefully, tucking in the ends. Serve with your favorite dipping sauce.

Quick Pad Thai

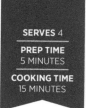

This traditional Thai stir-fried noodle dish cooks quickly, but all the prep work can make it seem laborious. Here, frozen stir-fry vegetables eliminate much of the work, making this tasty version come together much faster. Add more or less Sriracha depending on how spicy you like it.

1 POUND RICE NOODLES

1 PACKAGE (ABOUT 10 OUNCES) FROZEN STIR-FRY VEGETABLE MIX

1 TABLESPOON SESAME OIL

¼ CUP PURE MAPLE SYRUP

1 TABLESPOON SOY SAUCE

2 TABLESPOONS UNSEASONED RICE VINEGAR

1½ TEASPOONS TAMARIND PASTE

½ TO 1 TEASPOON SRIRACHA SAUCE (OR TO TASTE)

¼ CUP CHOPPED PEANUTS

1 CUP BEAN SPROUTS

1. Prepare the noodles according to package directions.

2. In a large skillet, heat the frozen vegetables over medium-high heat until warm, about 5 minutes.

3. Meanwhile, in a small bowl, stir together the sesame oil, maple syrup, soy sauce, vinegar, tamarind paste, and Sriracha. Add this sauce and the cooked noodles to the skillet with the vegetables and heat through. Serve topped with peanuts and bean sprouts.

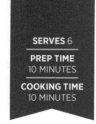
Seitan Gyro

Featuring all the classic flavors of gyro—tangy yogurt, pungent garlic, earthy oregano, and cumin—these pita sandwiches are sure to hit the spot. Add a helping of Red Onion Quick Pickle (page 71) for an extra-special treat.

1 ONION, DICED

1 CUCUMBER, DICED

1 CUP PLAIN SOY YOGURT

JUICE OF 1 LEMON

2 TABLESPOONS OLIVE OIL

1 POUND SEITAN, SHAVED INTO THIN PIECES

4 GARLIC CLOVES, MINCED

2 TEASPOONS DRIED OREGANO

1 TEASPOON GROUND CUMIN

6 PIECES PITA BREAD

1. In a small bowl, combine the onion, cucumber, yogurt, and lemon juice and refrigerate for 15 minutes.

2. In a medium pan, heat the olive oil over medium-high heat until it shimmers. Add the seitan, garlic, oregano, and cumin and cook until the seitan is cooked through, 7 to 10 minutes. Remove from the heat. Divide the seitan and cucumber mixture evenly, stuff them into six pitas, and serve immediately.

Chana Masala

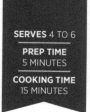

A Punjabi dish of chickpeas seasoned with garam masala (an Indian spice mixture containing pepper, cloves, cumin, and cardamom), this dish has a bright yellow color. Serve it over steamed rice or with naan bread for scooping and sopping up all the delicious sauce.

2 TABLESPOONS COCONUT OIL

1 ONION, DICED

5 GARLIC CLOVES, DICED

TWO 15-OUNCE CANS CHICKPEAS,
    DRAINED AND RINSED

JUICE OF 1 LEMON

2 TEASPOONS CURRY POWDER

1 TEASPOON GROUND CORIANDER

1 TEASPOON GARAM MASALA

1 CUP WATER

NAAN BREAD, FOR SERVING

1. In a large pot, heat the coconut oil over medium-high heat until it shimmers. Add the onion and cook until soft, about 5 minutes. Add the garlic and cook until it is fragrant, about 30 seconds.

2. Add the chickpeas, lemon juice, curry powder, coriander, garam masala, and water. Simmer, uncovered, stirring occasionally, until the chickpeas soften, about 10 minutes. Add more water if needed. Serve with naan.

Vegetable Biryani

Biryani typically calls for basmati rice, but using prepared white rice, along with frozen mixed vegetables, makes this an easy, fast weeknight meal. Serve it with a sauce of vegan yogurt raita with cucumbers.

1 PACKAGE (ABOUT 10 OUNCES)
   FROZEN MIXED VEGETABLES
3 TABLESPOONS COCONUT OIL
1 ONION, CHOPPED
2 GARLIC CLOVES, MINCED
½ TEASPOON GROUND TURMERIC

¼ TEASPOON GROUND CUMIN
¼ TEASPOON GROUND CORIANDER
¼ TEASPOON GROUND CINNAMON
2 TABLESPOONS GOLDEN RAISINS
4 CUPS PREPARED WHITE RICE

1. Cook the frozen vegetables according to package instructions. Set aside.

2. In a large pot, heat the coconut oil over medium-high heat until it shimmers. Add the onion and cook until soft, about 5 minutes. Add garlic, turmeric, cumin, coriander, and cinnamon and cook until they are fragrant, about 30 seconds. Add the raisins, rice, and vegetables and cook to heat through. Serve hot.

African Stew

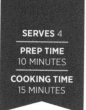

SERVES 4

PREP TIME
10 MINUTES

COOKING TIME
15 MINUTES

This hearty stew of tomatoes, yams, and the heady flavors of ginger and cayenne is enriched with peanut butter, which lends complexity and a pleasing creaminess to the dish. Be sure to use unsweetened yams.

Tip Instead of canned yams, use fresh ones. Prick them in several places with a fork, then microwave on high for 5 minutes or so until just tender. Peel and cut into large chunks before adding to the stew.

2 TABLESPOONS COCONUT OIL

1 ONION, CHOPPED

1 GREEN BELL PEPPER, CHOPPED

3 GARLIC CLOVES, MINCED

TWO 15-OUNCE CANS CHOPPED
   TOMATOES

1 CUP APPLE JUICE

TWO 15-OUNCE CANS UNSWEETENED
   YAMS, DRAINED

1 TEASPOON GROUND GINGER

¼ TEASPOON CAYENNE PEPPER

½ CUP CHUNKY PEANUT BUTTER

1. In a large pot, heat the coconut oil over medium-high heat until it shimmers. Add the onion and bell pepper and cook until they soften, about 5 minutes. Add the garlic and cook until it is fragrant, about 30 seconds.

2. Stir in the tomatoes, apple juice, yams, ginger, and cayenne and cook until heated through, about 5 minutes. Stir in the peanut butter and cook for another 5 minutes. Serve immediately.

Jamaican Jerk Tofu

Jerk seasoning is a mix of spices that includes allspice, nutmeg, cloves, and Scotch bonnet chiles. It can be found in the spice aisle of most grocery stores. Serve with a side of rice and some steamed vegetables.

Tip Jerk seasoning is available in the spice aisle of your supermarket, but it's simple to make at home. Combine ¼ cup brown sugar, 1 tablespoon allspice, 2 teaspoons dried thyme, 2 teaspoons salt, 1½ teaspoons cayenne pepper, 1 teaspoon freshly ground black pepper, ½ teaspoon ground nutmeg, ¼ teaspoon ground cinnamon, and ¼ teaspoon ground cloves. Store in an airtight container for up to 6 months.

2 TABLESPOONS JERK SEASONING

2 TABLESPOONS OLIVE OIL

1 POUND EXTRA-FIRM TOFU, PRESSED
    AND CUT INTO CUBES

2 TABLESPOONS COCONUT OIL

1 ONION, SLICED

1 ZUCCHINI, CHOPPED

1 CARROT, PEELED AND CHOPPED

1 GREEN BELL PEPPER, CHOPPED

3 GARLIC CLOVES, CHOPPED

1. In a small bowl, combine the jerk seasoning and olive oil.

2. In a medium bowl, add the tofu cubes and pour the olive oil and seasoning over the tofu. Refrigerate for at least 1 hour.

3. In a large sauté pan or wok, heat the coconut oil over medium-high heat until it shimmers. Add the onion, zucchini, carrot, and bell pepper and cook until the vegetables soften, about 5 minutes. Add the garlic and cook until it is fragrant, about 30 seconds. Stir in the tofu and cook until heated through, 2 to 3 minutes. Serve hot.

Enchiladas

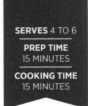

Chopped olives and onions make a hearty filling for these enchiladas. If you don't want to roll individual enchiladas, you can also make a casserole by layering sauce, tortillas, and filling and then topping with additional tortillas and sauce.

TWO 28-OUNCE CANS TOMATO SAUCE

1 TEASPOON DRIED OREGANO

2 TEASPOONS CHILI POWDER

2 TEASPOONS GARLIC POWDER

½ TEASPOON GROUND CUMIN

1 TABLESPOON OLIVE OIL

1 ONION, MINCED

THREE 2½-OUNCE CANS CHOPPED
   BLACK OLIVES

1 PACKAGE CORN TORTILLAS

1. Preheat the oven to 350°F. In a medium pot, heat the tomato sauce, oregano, chili powder, garlic powder, and cumin over medium-high heat until warmed through.

2. In a sauté pan, heat the olive oil until it shimmers. Add the onion and cook until soft, about 3 minutes. Remove from the heat and stir in the black olives.

3. In the bottom of a 13-by-9-inch baking dish, spread a thin layer of sauce. Dip each tortilla in the remaining sauce and place in the baking dish. Top each tortilla with onion and olives and roll. Pour the remaining sauce over the top. Bake for 15 minutes. Serve hot.

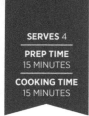
General Tso's Tofu

Ginger and garlic are the prominent flavors in this sweet and spicy tofu stir-fry, a takeoff on the well-known chicken dish. Serve it with Fried Rice (page 93) or with plain steamed rice.

Tip If you're avoiding soy, you can still enjoy this dish. Simply substitute seitan for the tofu and coconut aminos for the soy sauce. Both can be purchased at a health food or natural foods store.

3 TABLESPOONS COCONUT OIL

⅓ CUP PLUS 1½ TABLESPOONS
    CORNSTARCH

1 POUND EXTRA-FIRM TOFU, PRESSED
    AND CUT INTO CUBES

1 TABLESPOON GRATED FRESH GINGER

3 GARLIC CLOVES, MINCED

3 TABLESPOONS SOY SAUCE

1 TABLESPOON UNSEASONED
    RICE VINEGAR

¼ CUP AGAVE

1 CUP PLUS 2 TABLESPOONS
    VEGETABLE STOCK

1 TEASPOON RED PEPPER FLAKES
    (OR TO TASTE)

1. In a large sauté pan or wok, heat the coconut oil over medium-high heat until it shimmers. Put ⅓ cup of the cornstarch in a shallow bowl and dip the cubes of tofu into the cornstarch. Fry the tofu until golden brown, 3 to 4 minutes.

2. Meanwhile, in a small bowl, whisk together the ginger, garlic, soy sauce, vinegar, agave, 1 cup of the vegetable stock, and the red pepper flakes. Pour over the fried tofu in the pan and bring to a simmer.

3. In another small bowl, whisk together the remaining 1½ tablespoons cornstarch and 2 tablespoons vegetable stock to make a slurry. Add to the sauce and simmer until it thickens, 1 to 2 minutes. Serve hot.

Mushroom Paprikash

Choose sweet or hot paprika for this classic Eastern European dish. The sauce is a rich orange from the paprika and made creamy with vegan sour cream. Layer it atop rice or noodles to catch every bit of the saucy goodness.

2 TABLESPOONS OLIVE OIL

10 OUNCES SLICED CREMINI
    MUSHROOMS

1 ONION, MINCED

1 GREEN BELL PEPPER, MINCED

2 TABLESPOONS ALL-PURPOSE FLOUR

½ CUP WHITE WINE

2 TABLESPOONS PAPRIKA (EITHER
    SWEET OR HOT)

ONE 15-OUNCE CAN CRUSHED
    TOMATOES

¼ CUP VEGAN SOUR CREAM

1. In a large sauté pan, heat the olive oil over medium-high heat until it shimmers. Add the mushrooms and cook until they brown, about 7 minutes. Add the onion and bell pepper and cook until soft, about 3 minutes more.

2. Add the flour and cook, stirring constantly, for 2 minutes more. Add the wine and use a wooden spoon to scrape any browned bits off the bottom of the pan.

3. Add the paprika and tomatoes and cook until the sauce warms and thickens slightly, 3 to 4 minutes. Stir in the sour cream and serve immediately.

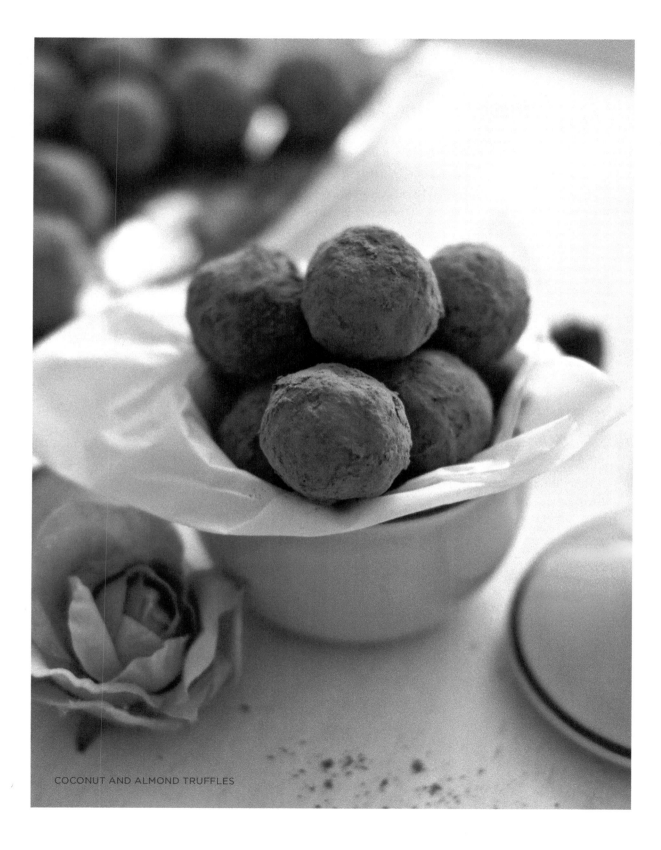

COCONUT AND ALMOND TRUFFLES

12

Desserts

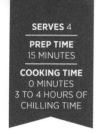

SERVES 4

PREP TIME
15 MINUTES

COOKING TIME
0 MINUTES
3 TO 4 HOURS OF
CHILLING TIME

Peach Sorbet

Peaches are the quintessential summer fruit, and sorbet is the perfect frozen treat for those hot summer days. This refreshing sorbet is easy to make. Use fresh, in-season peaches for best results. You can also replace the peaches with nectarines or berries.

5 PEACHES, PEELED, PITTED,
AND CHOPPED

¾ CUP SUGAR

JUICE OF 1 LEMON, OR 1 TABLESPOON
PREPARED LEMON JUICE

1. In the bowl of a food processor, combine all the ingredients and process until smooth.

2. Pour the mixture into a 9-by-13-inch glass pan. Cover tightly with plastic wrap. Freeze for 3 to 4 hours.

3. Remove from the freezer and scrape the sorbet into a food processor. Process until smooth. Freeze for another 30 minutes, then serve.

SERVES 4

PREP TIME
15 MINUTES

COOKING TIME
0 MINUTES
6 HOURS OF
CHILLING TIME

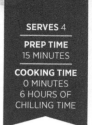

Lime and Watermelon Granita

Granita is a semi-frozen Italian dessert made with fresh fruit and sugar. The combination of lime juice and watermelon makes this version especially refreshing, but it can be made using just about any type of fruit.

Tip If you want to vary this granita, try adding a bit of grated fresh ginger or replace the lime juice with lemon or even grapefruit juice.

8 CUPS SEEDLESS
  WATERMELON CHUNKS
JUICE OF 2 LIMES, OR 2 TABLESPOONS
  PREPARED LIME JUICE

½ CUP SUGAR
STRIPS OF LIME ZEST, FOR GARNISH

1. In a blender or food processor, combine the watermelon, lime juice, and sugar and process until smooth. You may have to do this in two batches. After processing, stir well to combine both batches.

2. Pour the mixture into a 9-by-13-inch glass dish. Freeze for 2 to 3 hours.

3. Remove from the freezer and use a fork to scrape the top layer of ice. Leave the shaved ice on top and return to the freezer. In another hour, remove from the freezer and repeat. Do this a few more times until all the ice is scraped up. Serve frozen, garnished with strips of lime zest.

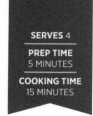
Chocolate Pudding

Who doesn't love a rich, creamy chocolate pudding? This dairy-free version is simple to make but no less delicious than the original. Be sure the cornstarch is whisked thoroughly into the almond milk to avoid lumpy pudding. You can top it with whipped coconut cream if you like.

Tip To make whipped coconut cream, refrigerate a can of full-fat coconut milk overnight and then spoon the thick cream that has risen to the top into a large bowl (save the milk for another purpose). Using an electric mixer set on high speed, whip the cream until it becomes very fluffy and forms soft peaks. Add a touch of honey or maple syrup if desired.

⅓ CUP SUGAR

⅓ CUP UNSWEETENED COCOA
   POWDER

3 CUPS UNSWEETENED ALMOND MILK

¼ CUP CORNSTARCH

PINCH OF SEA SALT

1 TEASPOON VANILLA EXTRACT

1. In a medium bowl, whisk together the sugar and cocoa powder to thoroughly combine. In a large saucepan over medium heat, whisk together the cocoa mixture and 2½ cups of the almond milk. Bring to a boil, stirring constantly. Remove from the heat.

2. In a small bowl, whisk together the remaining ½ cup almond milk and cornstarch. Stir into the cocoa mixture and return to medium heat. Add the salt.

3. Stirring constantly, bring the pudding to a boil. It will begin to thicken. Boil for 1 minute. Remove from the heat and stir in the vanilla. Chill before serving.

Peanut Butter and Crisped Rice Treats

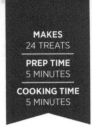

MAKES
24 TREATS

PREP TIME
5 MINUTES

COOKING TIME
5 MINUTES

Two childhood favorites—sweet crisped rice cereal bars and creamy, nutty peanut butter—come together here to create a dessert that is sure to make you feel like a kid again. It may be hard to wait to dig in, but it's important to chill it thoroughly before cutting it into pieces or you'll have a big mess on your hands (literally!).

Tip To make cleanup a snap, line the pan with parchment paper, leaving a bit hanging over the edge, before pouring in the hot cereal mixture. Once the mixture is completely chilled, it's easy to lift it out of the pan to cut into bars.

6 CUPS CRISPED RICE CEREAL
1 CUP CORN SYRUP

1 CUP SUGAR
1 CUP CHUNKY PEANUT BUTTER

1. Put the cereal in a large bowl. In a small saucepan, combine the corn syrup and sugar over medium-high heat. Cook, stirring constantly, until the mixture boils. Remove from the heat and stir in the peanut butter. Pour over the cereal and mix to combine.

2. Spread in a 9-by-13-inch pan. Chill for 1 hour and then cut into squares and serve.

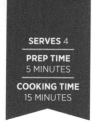
Caramelized Pears with Balsamic Glaze

A drizzle of tangy balsamic adds complexity to a dish of luscious caramelized pears. Use a good-quality aged balsamic vinegar for this dessert, as well as fresh pears that are ripe but not too soft. Bosc, Bartlett, or Asian pears work well here.

Tip You could substitute peaches, nectarines, or plums for a summery variation on this dish. Choose fruit that is ripe but still firm for best results.

1 CUP BALSAMIC VINEGAR

¼ CUP PLUS 3 TABLESPOONS
    BROWN SUGAR

¼ TEASPOON GRATED NUTMEG

PINCH OF SEA SALT

¼ CUP COCONUT OIL

4 PEARS, CORED AND CUT
    INTO SLICES

1. In a medium saucepan, heat the balsamic vinegar, ¼ cup of the brown sugar, the nutmeg, and salt over medium-high heat, stirring to thoroughly incorporate the sugar. Allow to simmer, stirring occasionally, until the glaze reduces by half, 10 to 15 minutes.

2. Meanwhile, heat the coconut oil in a large sauté pan over medium-high heat until it shimmers. Add the pears to the pan in a single layer. Cook until they turn golden, about 5 minutes. Add the remaining 3 tablespoons brown sugar and continue to cook, stirring occasionally, until the pears caramelize, about 5 minutes more.

3. Place the pears on a plate. Drizzle with balsamic glaze and serve.

Mixed Berries and Cream

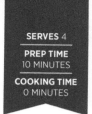

SERVES 4

PREP TIME
10 MINUTES

COOKING TIME
0 MINUTES

Ripe and colorful mixed berries with a touch of luscious, lightly sweetened cream make for a simple yet satisfying dessert. Use any combination of fresh berries you like for this dish. You can also zest a little orange over the top for even more flavor.

TWO 15-OUNCE CANS FULL-FAT
    COCONUT MILK
3 TABLESPOONS AGAVE
½ TEASPOON VANILLA EXTRACT

1 PINT FRESH BLUEBERRIES
1 PINT FRESH RASPBERRIES
1 PINT FRESH STRAWBERRIES, SLICED

1. Refrigerate the coconut milk overnight. When you open the can, the liquid will have separated from the solids. Spoon out the solids and reserve the liquid for another purpose.

2. In a medium bowl, whisk the agave and vanilla extract into the coconut solids. Divide the berries among four bowls. Top with the coconut cream. Serve immediately.

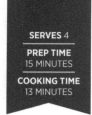

SERVES 4

PREP TIME
15 MINUTES

COOKING TIME
13 MINUTES

Spiced Apple Compote

Tender cooked apples sweetened with brown sugar, spiced with cinnamon, and topped with delightfully crunchy toasted pecans are like apple pie filling without the crust. For best results, choose sweet-tart apples like Granny Smith or Honeycrisp for this recipe.

Tip Top with a dollop of whipped coconut cream, if desired. To make whipped coconut cream, refrigerate a can of full-fat coconut milk overnight and then spoon the thick cream that has risen to the top into a large bowl (save the milk for another purpose). Using an electric mixer set on high speed, whip the cream until it becomes very fluffy and forms soft peaks. Add a touch of honey or maple syrup if desired.

4 SWEET-TART APPLES, CORED
   AND PEELED
½ CUP APPLE JUICE
JUICE OF 1 LEMON
¼ CUP BROWN SUGAR

¼ TEASPOON GRATED NUTMEG
1 TEASPOON GROUND CINNAMON
PINCH OF SEA SALT
½ CUP CHOPPED PECANS

1. In a saucepan, cook the apples, apple juice, lemon juice, brown sugar, nutmeg, cinnamon, and salt over medium-high heat, stirring occasionally, until the apples are tender, about 10 minutes. Remove from the heat and set aside.

2. Meanwhile, in a dry sauté pan over medium-high heat, toast the pecans, stirring frequently, about 3 minutes. Serve the compote warm topped with toasted pecans.

Spiced Rhubarb Sauce

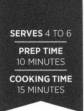

SERVES 4 TO 6

PREP TIME
10 MINUTES

COOKING TIME
15 MINUTES

While rhubarb is technically a vegetable, it functions as a fruit in this sweet-tart sauce. Serve it over vegan ice cream, layer it with vegan yogurt for a distinctive parfait, spoon it onto freshly baked biscuits, or use it as a sauce for fresh strawberries.

½ CUP WATER

½ CUP SUGAR

¼ TEASPOON GRATED NUTMEG

¼ TEASPOON GROUND GINGER

¼ TEASPOON GROUND CINNAMON

1 POUND RHUBARB, CUT INTO
  ½- TO 1-INCH PIECES

In a large saucepan, bring the water, sugar, nutmeg, ginger, and cinnamon to a boil. Add the rhubarb and cook over medium-high heat, stirring frequently, until the rhubarb is soft and saucy, about 10 minutes. Chill for at least 30 minutes before serving.

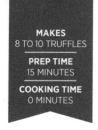

MAKES
8 TO 10 TRUFFLES

PREP TIME
15 MINUTES

COOKING TIME
0 MINUTES

Coconut and Almond Truffles

These silky, melt-in-your-mouth truffles are surprisingly easy to make. For variety in both flavor and appearance, roll the chocolate balls in any combination of unsweetened cocoa, chopped nuts, or unsweetened coconut flakes.

Tip This recipe is extremely versatile. Create different flavor combinations by adding coffee or mint extract, using hazelnut syrup in place of the maple syrup, or stirring warm spices like cinnamon, cloves, or even a touch of ground chile into the chocolate mixture.

1 CUP PITTED DATES

1 CUP ALMONDS

½ CUP SWEETENED COCOA POWDER,
    PLUS EXTRA FOR COATING

½ CUP UNSWEETENED SHREDDED
    COCONUT

¼ CUP PURE MAPLE SYRUP

1 TEASPOON VANILLA EXTRACT

1 TEASPOON ALMOND EXTRACT

¼ TEASPOON SEA SALT

1. In the bowl of a food processor, combine all the ingredients and process until smooth. Chill the mixture for about 1 hour.

2. Roll the mixture into balls and then roll the balls in cocoa powder to coat. Serve immediately or keep chilled until ready to serve.

Chocolate Macaroons

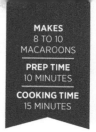

MAKES
8 TO 10
MACAROONS

PREP TIME
10 MINUTES

COOKING TIME
15 MINUTES

These chewy, chocolaty, and scrumptious macaroons require only a handful of ingredients and can be stirred together in just minutes. After a quick turn in the oven, you'll have an irresistible treat to satisfy your own cravings or to offer to guests after an elegant meal.

1 CUP UNSWEETENED SHREDDED
COCONUT

2 TABLESPOONS COCOA POWDER

⅔ CUP COCONUT MILK

¼ CUP AGAVE

PINCH OF SEA SALT

1. Preheat the oven to 350°F. Line a baking sheet with parchment paper. In a medium saucepan, cook all the ingredients over medium-high heat until a firm dough is formed.

2. Scoop the dough into balls and place on the baking sheet. Bake for 15 minutes, remove from the oven, and let cool on the baking sheet. Serve cooled macaroons or store in a tightly sealed container for up to 1 week.

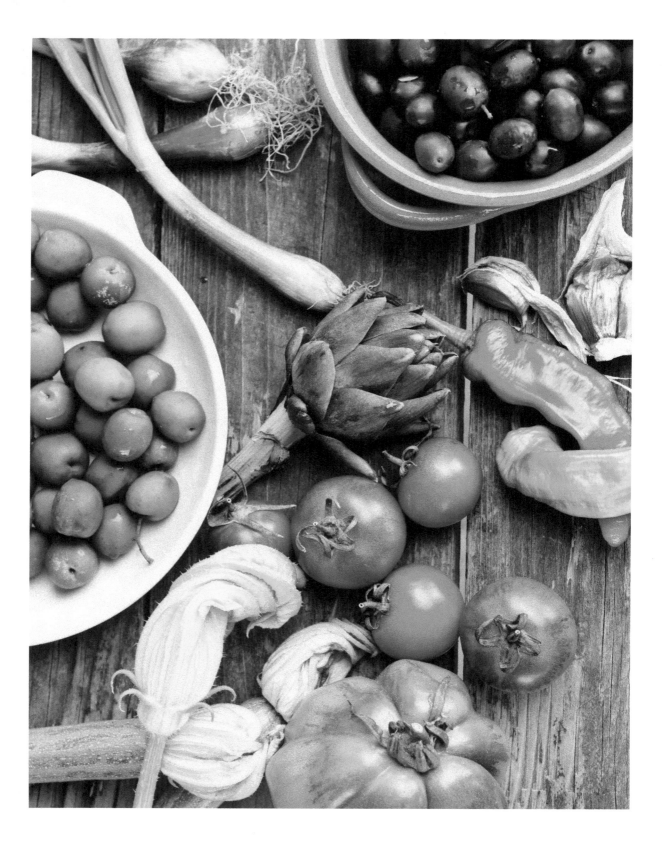

The Dirty Dozen and the Clean Fifteen

EATING CLEAN

Each year, Environmental Working Group, an environmental organization based in the United States, publishes a list they call the "Dirty Dozen." These are the fruits and vegetables that, when conventionally grown using chemical pesticides and fertilizers, carry the highest residues. If organically grown isn't an option for you, simply avoid these fruits and vegetables altogether. The list is updated each year, but here is the most recent list (2013).

Similarly, the Environmental Working Group publishes a list of "The Clean Fifteen," fruits and vegetables that, even when conventionally grown, contain very low levels of chemical pesticide or fertilizer residue. These items are acceptable to purchase conventionally grown.

You might want to snap a photo of these two lists and keep them on your phone to reference while shopping. Or you can download the Environmental Working Groups app to your phone or tablet.

THE DIRTY DOZEN

APPLE
STRAWBERRY
GRAPE
CELERY
PEACH
SPINACH
SWEET BELL
  PEPPER
IMPORTED
  NECTARINE
CUCUMBER
CHERRY TOMATO
SNAP PEA
POTATO

THE CLEAN FIFTEEN

ASPARAGUS
AVOCADO
CABBAGE
CANTALOUPE
CORN
EGGPLANT
GRAPEFRUIT
KIWI
MANGO
MUSHROOM
ONIONS
PAPAYA
PINEAPPLE
SWEET PEAS
  (FROZEN)
SWEET POTATO

UNIVERSAL

Conversion Charts

VOLUME EQUIVALENTS (LIQUID)		
U.S. STANDARD	U.S. STANDARD (OUNCES)	METRIC (APPROXIMATE)
2 TABLESPOONS	1 FL. OZ.	30 ML
¼ CUP	2 FL. OZ.	60 ML
½ CUP	4 FL. OZ.	120 ML
1 CUP	8 FL. OZ.	240 ML
1½ CUPS	12 FL. OZ.	355 ML
2 CUPS OR 1 PINT	16 FL. OZ.	475 ML
4 CUPS OR 1 QUART	32 FL. OZ.	1 L
1 GALLON	128 FL. OZ.	4 L

OVEN TEMPERATURES	
FAHRENHEIT (F)	CELSIUS (C) (APPROXIMATE)
250	120
300	150
325	165
350	180
375	190
400	200
425	220
450	230

VOLUME EQUIVALENTS (DRY)	
U.S. STANDARD	METRIC (APPROXIMATE)
⅛ TEASPOON	.5 ML
¼ TEASPOON	1 ML
½ TEASPOON	2 ML
¾ TEASPOON	4 ML
1 TEASPOON	5 ML
1 TABLESPOON	15 ML
¼ CUP	59 ML
⅓ CUP	79 ML
½ CUP	118 ML
⅔ CUP	156 ML
¾ CUP	177 ML
1 CUP	235 ML
2 CUPS OR 1 PINT	475 ML
3 CUPS	700 ML
4 CUPS OR 1 QUART	1 L
½ GALLON	2 L
1 GALLON	4 L

WEIGHT EQUIVALENTS	
U.S. STANDARD	METRIC (APPROXIMATE)
½ OUNCE	15 G
1 OUNCE	30 G
2 OUNCES	60 G
4 OUNCES	115 G
8 OUNCES	225 G
12 OUNCES	340 G
16 OUNCES OR 1 POUND	455 G

IN 30 MINUTES

Recipe Index

IN 30 MINUTES

Index

CPSIA information can be obtained
at www.ICGtesting.com
Printed in the USA
BVHW051532121219
566330BV00001B/1